High-Performance Membrane Dialyzers

Contributions to Nephrology

Vol. 173

Series Editor

Claudio Ronco Vicenza

High-Performance Membrane Dialyzers

Volume Editors

Akira Saito Isehara
Hideki Kawanishi Hiroshima
Akihiro C. Yamashita Fujisawa
Michio Mineshima Tokyo

61 figures, 7 in color, and 21 tables, 2011

KARGER Basel · Freiburg · Paris · London · New York · New Delhi · Bangkok · Beijing · Tokyo · Kuala Lumpur · Singapore · Sydney

Contributions to Nephrology
(Founded 1975 by Geoffrey M. Berlyne)

Akira Saito
Division of Nephrology and Metabolism
Department of Medicine
Tokai University School of Medicine
143 Shimokasuya
Isehara, Kanagawa, 259–1193 (Japan)

Hideki Kawanishi
Tsuchiya General Hospital
3-30 Nakajima-cho, Naka-ku
Hiroshima 730-8655 (Japan)

Akihiro C. Yamashita
Department of Human and Environmental Science, School of Engineering
Shonan Institute of Technology
1-1-25 Tsujido-Nishikaigan
Fujisawa, Kanagawa 251-8511 (Japan)

Michio Mineshima
Department of Clinical Engineering
Tokyo Women's Medical University
8-1, Kawada-cho, Shinjuku-ku
Tokyo 162-8666 (Japan)

Library of Congress Cataloging-in-Publication Data

High-performance membrane dialyzers / volume editors, Akira Saito ... [et al.].
p. ; cm. -- (Contributions to nephrology, ISSN 0302-5144 ; v. 173)
Includes bibliographical references and indexes.
ISBN 978-3-8055-9812-5 (hard cover : alk. paper) – ISBN 978-3-8055-9813-2 (e-ISBN)
1. Hemodialysis. 2. Blood–Filtration. 3. Membranes (Technology) I. Saito, Akira, 1943 Sept.-
II. Series: Contributions to nephrology ; v. 173. 0302-5144
[DNLM: 1. Hemodiafiltration–instrumentation. 2. Hemodiafiltration–methods. 3. Kidney, Artificial.
4. Membranes, Artificial. W1 CO778UN v.173 2011 / WJ 378]
RC901.7.H45H54 2011
617.4'61059--dc23

2011024148

Bibliographic Indices. This publication is listed in bibliographic services, including Current Contents® and Index Medicus.

www.karger.com
Printed in Switzerland on acid-free and non-aging paper (ISO 9706) by Reinhardt Druck, Basel
ISSN 0302–5144
ISBN 978–3–8055–9812–5
e-ISBN 978–3–8055–9813–2

Contents

Preface

by Akira Saito

Regenerated cellulose had been exclusively used as a dialysis membrane until the beginning of the 1980s since 1944, when Kolff et al. developed the drum-type dialysis system and used a cellophane membrane tube as a dialysis membrane. In the 1970s, synthetic membranes were used as hemofilters. In the 1970s, however, these membranes were not used as dialyzers because without a controller, an excess volume of water was removed from the body due to the characteristics of high-flux membranes. Therefore, a filtration volume controller was used instead in the 1980s, by which the ultrafiltration rate could be preset, thereby maintaining a stable ultrafiltration rate.

Middle molecular substances of 300–3,000 daltons were targeted for removal by hemodialysis and hemofiltration in the 1970s; this middle molecule removal was hypothesized by Babb et al. Despite testing the authenticity of the hypothesis for 10 years, researchers worldwide were unable to prove it. During and after this period, different directions in removal targets of uremic molecules were retrieved worldwide. Researchers in the USA focused on the kinetics of small molecular substances such as urea, and at the time the Kt/V value for urea was only used as a dialysis dose, whereas the researchers in Japan aimed at removing substances, ranging from small molecular substances to low molecular weight proteins, including small amounts of albumin, in order to approximate dialytic solute removal to glomerular filtration. Therefore, it is only in Japan that the specific name 'high-performance dialysis membrane (HPM)' is used for highly-permeable dialysis membranes with biocompatibility since the Japanese Society for HPM was established in 1985, and the First Annual Meeting for HPMs was held in Tokyo in 1986. HPM is different from 'highly permeable dialysis membranes' in that one of the solute removal characteristics of HPM is that it can remove a certain amount of albumin, which is also removed by glomerular filtration in the kidneys. Globally, except in Japan, small and middle molecular weight uremic toxins except albumin are the removal targets of hemodialysis. In 1997, HPMs were approved as type II dialyzers by the Japanese Government and were priced slightly higher than the conventional (type I) dialyzers. At that point, type II dialyzers were adjusted such that a clearance of β_2-microglobulin of more than 10 ml/min was obtained, whereas the type I dialyzers were adjusted such that the clearance of β_2-microglobulin was below the detectable level. Recently, the classification of dialyzers was revised from two types, i.e. I and II, to 5 types from I to V.

In this volume of *Contributions to Nephrology*, we have submitted 23 papers on HPM, which include the definition, kinetics of solutes, performances, clinical effects, and each characteristic of the HPMs. We are thankful for the opportunity to publish our papers titled 'High-Performance Dialysis Membranes' and receive opinions from researchers and physicians working on dialysis membranes worldwide.

We would like to thank the authors and all the contributors for the enormous effort and the quality of their scientific chapters. We would also like to thank all those who made this publication possible, in particular Karger Publishers.

Foreword

by Hideki Kawanishi

Dialyzers today are being developed towards high permeability and biocompatibility with an absolute need for solid evidence with regard to their abilities. High-flux dialyzers are recommended for the progress of good outcomes for dialysis populations. However, the definition of such high-flux dialyzers remains controversial. In Japan, the classification of dialyzers refers to five types, from I to V, that is they are classified for the clearance of β_2-microglobulin of less than 10, 30, 50, 70 and more than 70 ml/min at a blood flow rate of 200 ml/min and a dialyzer flow rate of 500 ml/min (see Appendix table). Especially types IV and V, the so-called 'super high-flux dialyzers', share over 90% of the market in Japan. The classification based on permeability is the simplest way of evaluating dialyzers. However, in order to clinically evaluate dialyzers, not only permeability but also biocompatibility should be taken into consideration. In Japan, the term 'high-performance membrane dialyzer (HPM dialyzer)' has in general been called so since 1985, and refers to both higher solute removal and good biocompatibility. The category of this type of HPM dialyzer, which has been developed by several manufacturers, is now appearing on the world market and is expected to improve the overall outcome of dialysis patients.

With the cooperation of the Japanese Society for HPM (JSHPM) and the Japanese Society for Hemodiafiltration (JSHDF), this issue of *Contributions to Nephrology* was planned in order to call attention to HPM dialyzers on a wider scale. We firmly believe that this book, the first of its kind specifically on the subject of HPM dialyzers, will be widely recommended for international guidelines in the future.

All authors and contributors are thanked for the enormous effort and high quality of their scientific papers. We also thank those who made this publication possible, in particular Karger Publishers.

Saito A, Kawanishi H, Yamashita AC, Mineshima M (eds): High-Performance Membrane Dialyzers.
Contrib Nephrol. Basel, Karger, 2011, vol 173, pp 1–10

Definition of High-Performance Membranes – From the Clinical Point of View

Akira Saito

Division of Nephrology and Metabolism, Department of Medicine, Tokai University School of Medicine, Isehara, and Division of Nephrology, Department of Medicine, Yokohama Dai-Ichi Hospital, Yokohama, Japan

Abstract

Global knowledge of the molecular target of uremic toxins (UTs) was significantly different in the 1980s than it is now. In 1971, Babb et al. hypothesized that UTs such as neurotoxin existed in mid-sized molecules ranging from 300 to 3,000 Da. In the 1980s, larger molecular weight substances >5,000 Da were targeted for removal, as well as small and medium size toxins in Japan, while urea was considered a surrogate marker of UTs, and Kt/V for urea was used as a measure of dialysis dose in the USA. In Japan, albumin-bound toxins in addition to low-molecular-weight proteins were targeted for removal as glomerular filtration in the normal kidney. As binding capacity of albumin is significantly lowered and, on the other hand, the α-helical content of albumin also lowered in uremic patients because of binding of UTs to albumin, a small amount of albumin should be removed to stimulate the synthesis of new albumin. KF101 C-2 (EVAL) used as a high-performance dialysis membrane (HPM) at the first step, in which approximately 7 g of albumin is removed per dialysis session. It resulted in lowered plasma albumin levels in hemodialysis patients, although accumulated levels of low-molecular-weight proteins were significantly lowered. Therefore, the Japanese Society of Dialysis Therapy has recommended limitation of albumin removal to <3 g/session by the second generation of HPMs. Many different HPMs have been developed since the Japanese Society of HPM was first organized in 1985. Approximately 98% of the dialyzers used in Japan employ HPMs. New technology is required to suppress fouling on the surface and in the pores of HPMs. This would maintain permeation of inflammatory cytokines during dialysis sessions.

The first dialysis membranes used in hemodialysis (HD) were regenerated cellulosic membranes (RCs). Such membranes have almost the same diameter of the pore which is relatively small. Originally, the molecular targets for diffusive removal in HD were small molecules, which were small enough to be removed by dialysis membrane made of cellulose. By 1970, it was considered that essentially all uremic toxins (UTs) were small molecules such as urea, creatinine, uric acid, methylguanidine. At that time, RCs were considered suitable for HD treatment of patients with renal failure not only in terms of the efficacy of removal of small molecular UTs, but also the strength of the membrane against the physical power for the construction of Kiil dialyzer in dialysis units [1].

However, in 1971, it was hypothesized that increased removal of larger molecular weight UTs than UTs indicated in the 1960s was important for the improvement of remaining complications such as uremic neuropathy in patients on HD [2, 3]. Beginning in 1973, efforts were initiated to improve the biocompatibility of dialysis membranes to avoid the stimulation of complement activation, as a result of interactions of the membrane with blood cells and biologically active plasma proteins [4, 5]. Synthetic membranes, as well as modified cellulose membrane such as cellulose acetate, have become widely accepted since 1985.

Highly permeable dialysis membranes with improved biocompatibility were produced by several companies in Japan in the 1980s. These membranes are known as 'HPMs' – high-performance dialysis membranes. These membrane modules have been actively evaluated in basic and clinical research. HPMs, therefore, are currently used in 98.3% treatments of HD patients in Japan [6]. In this paper the author describes the definition, developmental history, clinical evaluation, and future perspectives related to development of HPM.

Definition of an HPM

In order for the efficacy of removal characteristic of UTs in HD or hemofiltration (HF) to approach to glomerular filtration of the human kidney, the Japanese Society for Dialysis Therapy (JSDT) recommended that the pore size of HPM should be larger than the common pore size of conventional HD and HF membranes. This would allow permeation of medium and large molecules, including low-molecular-weight proteins (LMWPs) and a small amount of albumin [7]. The JSDT recommended that a small amount of albumin, ↓ <3 g/session under the conditions of blood flow rate at 200 ml/min, dialysate flow rate at 500 ml/min should be removed because the removal would induce an acceleration of turnover of albumin and considerable amounts of LMWPs such as β_2-microglobulin, and inflammatory cytokines, as well as sufficient removal of small molecular substances. In addition, it was recognized that membrane biocompatibility was required to avoid activation of the complement system, to prevent adhesion of proteins and blood cells including red blood cells and platelets onto the membrane surface, to prevent production of radicals from neutrophils, and to avoid generating advanced glycation end products. These issues were problematic with conventional RC membranes.

History of Development of Dialysis Membranes Since the 1970s

In the 1960s, most dialysis membranes used throughout the world were made of RC. These membranes were used as plate membranes in Kiil dialyzers [1] or coil dialyzers [8], because the RC dialysis membrane was generally considered to be economical, and capable of withstanding the physical power in constructing the dialyzers. This type of membrane had relatively small pores with even diameters and high densities that enabled sufficient clearance of small UTs. In 1971, Babb et al. [2] hypothesized that additional UTs, including peripheral neurotoxins, exist among the UTs with mid-range molecular weights. This concept was based on the low incidence of neuropathy in patients with renal failure treated with peritoneal dialysis. It was thought that in this type of dialysis higher clearance of mid-sized molecules contributed to the low incidence of the neuropathy, although the clearance of urea nitrogen was lower than that obtained with HD. They suggested that a square meter of dialysis membrane × dialysis time (hours) was positively correlated with high clearance of mid-sized molecules [2], ranging from 300 to 3,000 Da [3]. Therefore, clearance of molecules with higher molecular weights was considered to be obtained from dialysis performed using a membrane with a larger area and a longer treatment time than that used in conventional dialysis at that time.

This hypothesis was aggressively and globally investigated by many researchers in the 1970s. On the other hand, Henderson et al. [9, 10] investigated a combined therapy with HD and HF, which became known as diafiltration. HF was first applied clinically to treatment of renal failure patients with severe complications such as hypertension [11]. This treatment was based on the development of hemofilters that allow clearance of mid-sized molecular UTs to a greater extent than HD. However, no mid-sized UT was identified and the clinical significance of removal of mid-sized molecules was not clarified at that time. At the beginning of the 1980s, the number of studies on removal of mid-sized molecules and the clinical effects of HF declined remarkably.

In the 1980s, in the United States, the leading researchers became convinced that UTs did not exist in the middle molecular weight range. These researchers eventually focused on studies of urea kinetics and the use of the urea Kt/V value as a marker to quantify dialysis adequacy [12, 13] instead of identification and removal of mid-sized UTs. During this time, I suspected that larger molecular UTs might be present in uremic patients, and that the molecular weights of these molecules were not within the range of 300–5,000 Da.

Basic Concept of HPMs

Severe complications such as dialysis-related amyloidosis increased with dialysis time in long-term HD patients in Japan in the 1980s. This occurred even if patients received HD with sufficient clearance of small molecules. We suspected that either mid-sized molecular UTs ranging from 300 to 3,000 Da had not been sufficiently removed by HF with hemofilters produced in the 1970s, or that molecular UTs >5,000 Da should be targeted for removal from the blood of dialysis patients in order to prevent the onset and progression of these complications. In addition to small molecular substances, LMWPs including small amounts of albumin are filtered across the glomerular basement membrane, and a slit diaphragm is formed by the foot processes of podocytes. Albumin was detected in glomerular filtrate obtained from intraluminal fluid of proximal tubules using the micropuncture method [14]. I was convinced that this is not due to a kidney defect, instead it indicates an essential role of glomerular filtration in removing albumin-bound UTs. The albumin incorporated into tubular epithelial cells is degraded into amino acids and peptides by tubular proteases, and the amino acids and peptides are reabsorbed into the blood. Considerable amounts of LMWPs and some grams of albumin filtered daily from the glomerulus are reabsorbed as amino acids and peptides, because these proteins should be replaced by newly synthesized proteins that would be more effective in binding newly produced UTs or physiologically active substances. Proteins removed by dialysis using HPMs, however, cannot be recovered because the reabsorptive function of renal tubules is lacked in HD system. Therefore, the same amount of albumin cannot be removed on a weekly basis as would be removed by a normally functioning glomerulus. We decided to test the clinical significance of removal of albumin and LMWPs using several new dialyzers and filters with several levels of sieving coefficients of albumin and LMWPs [15–21]. SDS-polyacrylamide gel electrophoresis patterns of ultrafiltrates obtained using HPMs constructed between 1981 and 1984 are shown in figure 1.

Clinical Evaluation of HD Treatments Using HPMs in the 1980s

First Step of Development of HPMs

In a first step toward development of HPMs approaching the efficiency of glomerular filtration, I first collaborated with Kuraray Company to develop an ethylene vinyl alcohol copolymer (EVAL) membrane with an appropriate pore size in 1981, with the objective of removing considerable amounts of albumin and LMWPs. EVAL membrane KF101 C-2 was evaluated as a hemofilter and C-2B was evaluated as a hemodialyzer between 1982 and 1986 [15–19]. Although large amounts of albumin were removed by hemodiafiltration using EVAL KF101 C-2, considerable amounts of LMWPs were also removed as 'protein-permeable hemodiafiltration', and clinical symptoms and complications including renal anemia, pruritus, pigmentation, and joint pain induced by β_2- microglobulin amyloidosis [22] were improved. Saito et al. [19] reported a cross-over clinical trial using KF101-C-2B and RC dialyzers, AM-20 (Asahi

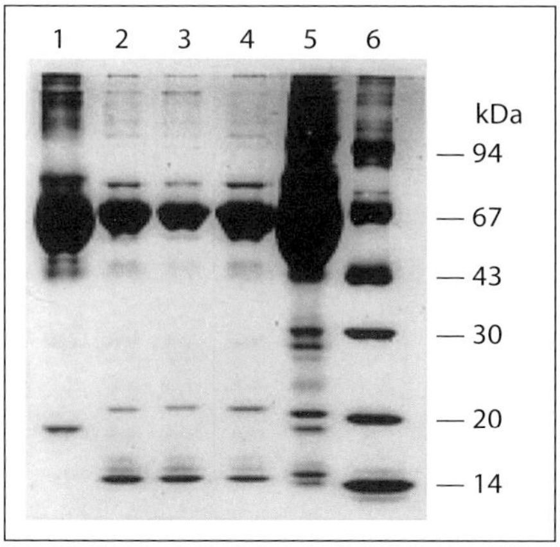

Fig. 1. Electrophoretic patterns of filtrate obtained from plasma of a uremic patient across six kinds of HPM: 1 = TK-401, 2 = TAF-80S, 3 = Duo-Flux HP, 4 = TAF-120S, 5 = C-2, 6 = standard sample. Polymethylmethacrylate TK-401 membrane was from Toray Co., Tokyo, regenerated cellulose TAF-80S,120S from Terumo Co., Tokyo, cellulose diacetate Duo-Flux HP from CD Medical Int. Ltd, Miami Lake, Fla., USA, and ethylene vinyl alcohol (EVAL) copolymer C-2 from Kuraray Co., Kurashiki. Although considerable amounts of albumin and LMWPs were obtained with TK-401 and EVAL C-2 at the first step of development of HPM, albumin removal was suppressed with TAF and Duo-Flux HP membranes at the second step.

Chemical Co., Tokyo, Japan) over a 4-month period. Although removal of albumin and LMWPs in patients treated with RC was negligible, it became apparent that significant amounts of LMWPs were being removed by HD with the EVAL C-2B dialyzer. Hemoglobin levels in patients treated with the EVAL C-2B were significantly higher than in patients treated with AM-20 dialyzers. Table 1A and B provide a comparison of weekly removal of albumin and several LMWPs as well as plasma levels of these proteins before and 1 year after the start of each treatment in patients treated with dialysis using the EVAL C-2B membrane and patients treated with CAPD using 1.5% dextrose containing Dianeal PD fluid (Baxter Co., Alton, Ill., USA) 2 liters 3 times and a single treatment with 2 liters of 4.25% dextrose, with a total of 4 exchanges daily.

Before initiation of the study, all patients were treated by HD with conventional RC membrane dialyzer AM-20. Clinical improvement of renal anemia was also seen in patients treated with C-2B, because the middle molecular weight inhibitor of erythropoiesis that affects erythroid colony formation was removed by HPM (fig. 2) [23]. Small molecular inhibitors such as spermine were also removed [24]. However, plasma levels of albumin were significantly lower 1 year after the start of HD treatment than before the treatment in patients treated with KF101 C-2B, because the amount of albumin removed was presumed to be as much as 7 g/session and 22 g/week. The amounts of LMWPs and albumin

Table 1. Comparison of weekly removal of proteins by CAPD and HD with HPM

A Weekly removal of proteins

Proteins	Molecular weight Da	CAPD (n = 10) mg/week	HD with HPM (n = 10) mg/week
β_2-Microglobulin	11,800	229.5±31.4	246.7±26.1
Retinol-binding protein	21,000	180.2±30.6	232.5±42.1
α_1-Acidic glycoprotein	40,000	896.4±206.4	855.9±189.4
β_2-Glycoprotein 1	40,000	147.3±29.4	152.4±40.8
α_2-HS-glycoprotein	49,000	259.6±164.5	368.7±162.2
α_2-Antitrypsin	54,000	1,766.1±351.4	1,896.2±412.7
Prealbumin	55,000	192.6±54.8	248.4±50.8
Hemopexion	57,000	390.9±67.2	478.2±86.6
Albumin	67,000	18,673.2±3,654.3	22,365.0±3,759.6
Transferrin	76,000	1,252.8±368.4	1,430.4±540.9

B Plasma proteins in patients treated before and 1 year after each treatment

Plasma proteins	CAPD, mg/dl		HD with HPM		Normal range mg/dl
	n = 12	n = 12	n = 12	n = 12	
β_2-Microglobulin	5.1±2.0	3.7±1.5	6.0±1.6	4.8±1.5[1]	0.08–0.24
Retinol-binding protein	23.8±3.7	23.6±6.3	31.8±5.6	27.5±8.2	3–6
α_1-Acidic glycoprotein	127.6±44.4	148.6±49.6	94.1±36.6	103.7±40.8	40–80
β_2-Glycoprotein-1	32.3±2.5	38.1±8.5	29.6±5.1	31.6±6.0	10–20
α_2-HS-glycoprotein	64.2±13.1	78.1±18.8	57.5±5.0	50.8±5.4	30–70
α_1-Antitrypsin	149.3±28.8	156.4±48.6	133.8±30.6	150.0±40.1	170–360
Prealbumin	40.1±5.0	42.2±11.7	43.3±7.6	39.2±6.8	12–28
Hemopexin	73.1±6.0	70.0±13.8	76.3±10.6	68.5±12.1	40–60
Albumin	3500±410	3720±508	4220±521	3601±597[2]	3,500–5,000
Transferrin	191.1±57.1	247.9±67.4[1]	202.8±51.9	242.3±56.8[2]	210–290

[1] $p < 0.01$, compared to values before the treatment.
[2] $p < 0.05$, compared to values before the treatment.

removed weekly from HD patients treated with the KF101 C-2B dialyzer were somewhat larger than those removed from patients treated with CAPD.

After clinical evaluation of the first generation of HPMs, we submitted requests to dialyzer companies for development of new dialysis membranes to suppress the sieving coefficient (SC) of albumin by <0.03 while maintaining the SC of LMWPs >0.5 under the filtration rate at 10 ml/min at the first 30 min of treatment in 1983. Albumin removal by the TAF-120S dialyzer was apparently

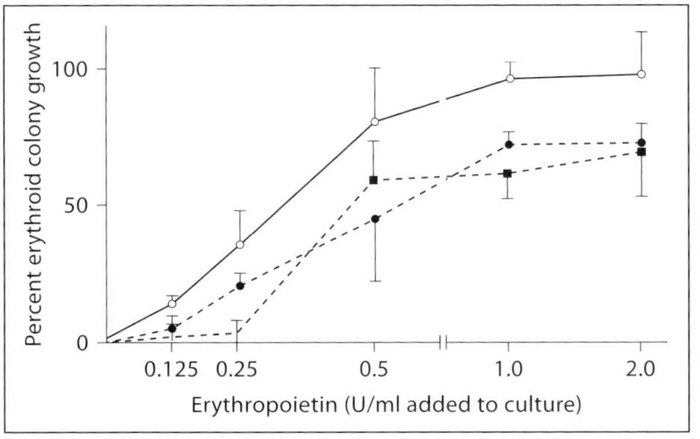

Fig. 2. Inhibitory effect of spermine and the middle molecular weight inhibitor of erythropoiesis on the number of mouse erythroid colonies with doses of erythropoietin added to the culture medium. Middle molecular weight inhibitor of erythropoiesis added was obtained from a fraction collected by ion exchange chromatography with a DEAE Sephadex A-25 column. This fraction was collected from the middle molecular fraction of gel filtration with Sephadex G-50. The percent erythroid colony growth was lowered, when spermine (+) or the middle molecular inhibitor of erythropoiesis (I) was added to the culture, in comparison with that in control (y), regardless of the doses of erythropoietin.

lowered <3 g/session [25]. We organized the Japanese Society for HPM in 1985 and its first meeting was held in Tokyo in 1986. Additional HPM dialyzers, which included other synthetic membranes such as polysulfone, polyacrylonitrile, and other membranes, were developed from 1985 to 1990.

Advantages and Disadvantages of Albumin Removal

Although dialysis membranes are produced to avoid permeation of albumin, we wished to develop HPMs that allow albumin to permeate at a rate of <3 g/session [7] and approximately <1.7 g/day. This would prevent plasma albumin levels from being significantly lowered in dialysis patients treated with HPMs. Albumin-binding UTs are filtered through the glomerular basement membrane and slit diaphragm and incorporated into tubule cells and degraded into amino acids that are absorbed into the blood while UTs were passed into the urine. There are several binding sites in the hydrophobic and hydrophilic portions of the three-dimensional structure of albumin. Binding sites of albumin are occupied by specific toxins or several nonspecific UTs in uremic patients. The three-dimensional structure of albumin, from a different point of view, was confirmed to be changed in uremia. The α-helical content of uremic albumin in uremic filtrate except proteins was found to be remarkably decreased [26], as indicated by observing the negative UV peak at 222 nm in the circular dichroism spectrum (table 2) [27]. Albumin is important in terms of not only its concentration in plasma but also its functional capacity for binding to toxins. Aged albumin,

Table 2. α-Helical contents of albumin detected by the negative UV peak at 222 nm in the circular dichroism spectrum

Albumin obtained from	Solvent liquid of albumin solution	α-Helix content at 222 nm (m^2)
Normal subjects (n = 6)	PBS	10.01±0.43
Regular dialysis patients (n = 10)	PBS	9.92±1.05
	ultrafiltrate from serum of regular dialysis patients	9.1±1.04
Severe uremic patients (n = 6)	PBS	9.66±1.53
	ultrafiltrate from	7.48±1.72

Cell size: 0.5 mm; concentration of albumin solution: 30 mg/dl; PBS = phosphate-buffered saline.

in which various UTs are bound to essentially all binding sites in the hydrophobic and hydrophilic portions of the three-dimensional structure, should be exchanged, or regenerated, therefore an appropriate amount of albumin should be removed to produce new albumin.

A disadvantage of removing albumin with HD using HPMs is that >9 g of albumin would be removed on a weekly basis. However, albumin synthesis would be accelerated in the liver by the feedback mechanism. Low levels of albumin are well recognized as a mortality risk. However, mortality is correlated with low serum albumin only as a result of malnutrition and/or oxidative and inflammatory states. Lowered albumin levels induced by dialysis have not been demonstrated to be a risk factor for mortality.

Future Perspectives on the Development of HPMs

Current HPMs are not ideal. HPMs capable of filtering relatively high-molecular-weight LMWPs such as interleukin (IL)-1, IL-6 and tumor necrosis factor-α should also have the ability to suppress removal of albumin to <3 g/session. A significant difference in removal of albumin and LMWPs has not been reached in current dialysis membrane technology. In order to modify current HD treatment to allow HD patients to survive for a long duration, we must overcome the problem of chronic inflammation induced by endotoxin-contaminated dialysis fluid, bioincompatible dialyzers, and uremia itself. Therefore, all dialysis components such as ultrapure and acetate-free dialysate, biocompatible dialysis membranes, and combined use of diffusion and convection to remove a wide range of substances from small to mid-sized molecules have been recently employed. Since dialysis purity has improved and biocompatible dialysis membranes have been developed over the past two decades, the incidence of surgery to treat carpal tunnel syndrome has been lowered in cases of β_2-microglobulin amyloidosis [28, 29]. However, removal of LMWPs, such as IL-1, IL-6, tumor necrosis factor-α with molecular weights ranging from 15,000 to 25,000 Da, were considered insufficient to prevent long-term complications, such as atherosclerosis, cardiovascular diseases, malnutrition and β_2-microglobulin amyloidosis. It is also difficult to employ dialysis to remove relatively large molecular weight LMWPs such as inflammatory cytokines. Such proteins cause biofouling by becoming adsorbed onto the surface and inside the pores of the membranes during the HD treatment. As a result of fouling, removal of inflammatory cytokines decreases remarkably during the first hour of treatment. We should clarify the detailed mechanism of the biofouling phenomenon and characterize the fouling behavior of each dialysis membrane. New anti-biofouling technology should be developed over the course of the next decade to precisely control the amounts of albumin and inflammatory cytokines removed in each dialysis session. This will prevent the progression of chronic inflammation in patients undergoing long-term dialysis.

References

1 Kiil F: Development of a parallel-flow artificial kidney in plastics. Acta Chir Scand 1960;253(suppl):142–150.

2 Babb AL, Popovich RP, Christopher TG, Scribner BH: The genesis of the square meter-hour hypothesis. Trans Am Soc Artif Intern Organs 1971;7:81–86.

3 Babb AL, Farrell PC, Uvelli DA, Scribner BH: Hemodialyzer evaluation by examination of solute molecular spectra. Trans Am Soc Artif Intern Organs 1972;18:98–101.

4 Craddock PR, Fehr J, Dalmasso AP, Brighan KL, Jacob HS: Hemodialysis leucopenia: pulmonary vascular leukostasis resulting from complement activation by dialyzer cellophane membranes. J Clin Invest 1977;59: 879–888.

5 Chenoweth DE: Complement activation during hemodialysis: clinical observations, proposed mechanisms and theoretical implications. Artif Organs 1984;8:281–287.

6 Statistics Committee of the Japanese Society of Dialysis Therapy: Illustration. Present status of maintenance dialysis in Japan on December 31, 2008 (in Japanese). J Jap Soc Dial Ther 2009:30–38.

7 Kolff WJ, Wàtschinger B: Further development of a coil kidney. Disposable artificial kidney. J Lab Clin Med 1956;47:969–977.

8 Sato T, Saito A, Naito H, Yamagami S, Akizawa T, Akiba T, Takezawa S: Function and adaptation of blood purification methods. Evaluation methods and functional classification of dialyzers and hemofilters (in Japanese). J Jap Soc Dial Ther 1996;29:1231–1245.

9 Henderson LW, Livoti LG, Ford CA, Kelly AB, Lysaght MJ: Clinical experience with intermittent hemodiafiltrations. Trans Am Soc Artif Intern Organs 1973;19:119–123.

10 Henderson LW, Silverstein ME, Ford CA, Lysaght MJ: Clinical response to maintenance hemodiafiltration. Kidney Int 1975;7(suppl):58–62.

11 Quellhorst E, Rieger J, Doht B: Treatment of chronic uremia by an ultrafiltration kidney – first clinical experience. Proc Eur Dial Transplant Assoc 1976;13:314–317.

12 Lowrie EG, Laird NM, Parker TF, Sargent JA: Effect of the hemodialysis prescription on patient morbidity: report from the National Cooperative Dialysis Study. N Engl J Med 1981;305:1176–1181.

13 Gotch F, Sargent JA: A mechanistic analysis of the National Cooperative Dialysis Study. Kidney Int 1985;28:526–534.

14 Leber PD, Marsh DJ: Micropuncture study of concentration and fate of albumin in rat nephron. Am J Physiol 1970;219:358–363.

15 Saito A, Chung TG, Kanazawa I, Oda O, Ohta K: Clinical evaluation of protein permeating hemofilter and analysis of middle molecules in ultrafiltrate (in Japanese). Jinkou-Zouki 1981;10:907–911.

16 Saito A, Chung TG, Kanazawa I, Ogawa H, Ohta K: Middle and large molecule removal of protein-permeating hemodiafiltration; in Piskin E, Chang TMS (eds): Proc 4th Int Symp Hemoperfusion Artif Organs. Ankara, Turkish Artificial Organs Society, 1982, pp 42–46.

17 Saito A, Ogawa H, Takagi H, Chung TG: Clinical effects of large molecule removal by protein-permeable hemofilters (in Japanese). Jin to Touseki 1983;15:767–772.

18 Saito A, Ogawa H, Takagi H, Chung TG: Clinical evaluation of protein-permeating hemodiafiltration (in Japanese). Jinkou-Zouki 1984;13:643–646.

19 Saito A, Naito H, Hirohata M: Dialytic removal of middle molecules and low molecular weight proteins; in Atsumi K, Maekawa M, Ota K (eds): Progress in Artificial Organs. Cleveland, ISAO Press, 1984, pp 412–416.

20 Saito A, Ogawa H, Chung TG, Maeda K: CAPD and protein-permeating hemodialysis: a clinical comparison; in Maher JF, Winchester JF (eds): Frontiers in Peritoneal Dialysis. New York, Field, Rich & Assoc Inc, 1986, pp 307–311.

21 Saito A, Ogawa H, Tkagi H, Ohta K, Akasu H, Kawai S, Kubotsu A: A new approach to glomerular filtration. Trans Am Soc Artif Intern Organs 1983;29:673–677.

22 Gejyo F, Yamada T, Odani S, Nakagawa Y, Arakawa M, Kunitomo T, Kataoka H, Suzuki M, Hirasawa Y, Shirahama T: A new form of amyloid protein associated with hemodialysis was identified as β_2-microglobulin. Biochem Biophys Res Commun 1985,129:701–706.

23 Saito A, Suzuki I, Chung TG, Ogawa, Ohta K: Separation of an inhibitor of erythropoiesis in 'middle molecules' from hemodialysate from patients with chronic renal failure. Clin Chem 1986;32:1938–1941.

24 Saito A, Takagi T, Chung TG, Ohta K: Serum levels of polyamines in patients with chronic renal failure. Kidney Int 1983;24(suppl 16): S234–S237.

25 Takagi T, Taoka M, Sakurai K, Ogawa H, Saito A: Removal of low molecular weight proteins by hemodialysis with several kinds of high-performance membrane dialyzers (in Japanese). Jin to Touseki 1987;86(suppl): 8–11.

26 Saito A, Yamamoto Y, Maeda K, Kobayashi K, Ohta K: Abnormal conformation of albumin in uremia. Proc Eur Dial Transpl Assoc 1978;15:628–629.

27 Saito A: Conformational change of albumin in uremia (in Japanese). Rinsho-Kagaku 1979;7:249–254.

28 Koda Y, Nishi S, Miyazaki S, Haginoshita S, Sakurabayashi T, Suzuki M, Sakai S, Yuasa Y, Hirasawa Y, Nishi T: Switch from conventional to high-flux membrane reduces the risk of carpal tunnel syndrome and mortality of hemodialysis patients. Kidney Int 1997;52: 1096–1101.

29 Schwalbe S, Holzhauer M, Schaeffer J, Galanski M, Koch KM, Floege J: Beta-2-microglobulin-associated amyloidosis: a vanishing complication of long-term hemodialysis? Kidney Int 1997;52:1077–1083.

Akira Saito, MD, PhD
Division of Nephrology and Metabolism
Department of Medicine, Tokai University School of Medicine
143, Shimokasuya, Isehara, Kanagawa 259-1193 (Japan)
Tel. +81 463 93 1121, E-Mail asait@is.icc.u-tokai.ac.jp

Saito A, Kawanishi H, Yamashita AC, Mineshima M (eds): High-Performance Membrane Dialyzers.
Contrib Nephrol. Basel, Karger, 2011, vol 173, pp 11–22

Solute Removal Efficiency and Biocompatibility of the High-Performance Membrane – From Engineering Points of View

Kiyotaka Sakai · Masato Matsuda

Department of Chemical Engineering, Waseda University, Tokyo, Japan

Abstract

Two major prerequisites of high-performance dialysis membranes are superior biocompatibility and high removal efficiency of pathogenic substances of large molecular size. In this article, we present a review, in the context of recent research results, of the solute removal efficiency and biocompatibility of the high-performance membrane. The former is discussed in terms of differences in separation properties arising from the constituent materials, the dialysis membrane structures, internal filtration-accelerated dialyzers, optimization of the dialysis fluid flow, and solute removal by adsorption, and the latter in terms of invasion of endotoxins present in dialysis fluid, antioxidant actions, and properties of the internal surface of dialysis membranes. We also discuss the main properties and problems of currently available high-performance dialysis membranes. While the solute removal efficiency of high-performance dialysis membranes is already mostly satisfactory and no further significant improvements are expected, except in relation to the fractioning properties (selectivity), there is much scope for improvement in the biocompatibility of dialysis membranes. It is important that ultrahigh-performance dialysis membranes of superior biocompatibility are developed based on the results of basic studies carried out from the engineering point of view, reports from the manufacturers, and clinical outcomes.

Ever since β_2-microglobulin was identified as the substance associated with dialysis-related amyloidosis, a well-known dialysis-related complication, earnest attempts have been made to increase the diameter of pores in dialysis membranes, for efficient removal of low-molecular-weight proteins, including

β_2-microglobulin [1, 2]. Because the problem of leakage of useful proteins, such as albumin, would then arise during dialysis, dialysis membranes with a sharp fractioning efficiency (selectivity) and optimized pore size distribution are developed to prevent leakage of albumin while still allowing removal of pathogenic low-molecular-weight proteins at a high efficiency [3]. Such dialysis membranes are referred to as high-performance dialysis membranes. However, even with the use of high-performance dialysis membranes, it is not always possible to entirely prevent complications associated with long-term dialysis and development of fever, inflammation, pain, or itching during dialysis treatment [4]. Thus, there is still need for further improvement of the fractioning efficiency of pathogenic substances and also of the biocompatibility of currently available high-performance dialysis membranes. Polysulfone (PSf) dialysis membranes, among the high-performance dialysis membranes that show superior biocompatibility and solute permeability, and allow control of the membrane pore size tailored to individual patients, have been gaining in popularity recently [5]. To obtain favorable solute permeability and favorable biocompatibility of high-performance dialysis membranes, basic studies at the micro- and nano-levels are needed, for example on the optimal diameter of the pores in the membrane and properties of the internal surface, and also basic studies at the macro-level, for example, investigation of the shape of the dialyzer jacket and the method of filling the dialysis membrane. In this article, we present a review of high-performance dialysis membranes from the engineering standpoint, focusing on the mechanisms/properties underlying the superior performance of the currently available high-performance dialysis membranes, and also discuss the problems that need to be overcome, in the light of results obtained from recent studies.

Solute Removal Efficiency

Difference in Separation Properties Arising from the Material(s) Constituting the Membrane Structure

Dialyzers can be classified as coil-, laminate-, and hollow-fiber-type dialyzers, and most dialyzers currently in use are hollow-fiber-type dialyzers. The materials most widely used at present for the manufacture of dialysis membranes are PSf, polyether sulfone (PES), and cellulose triacetate (CTA), besides polymethylmethacrylate (PMMA), polyester polymer alloys (PEPA), ethylene vinyl alcohol copolymers (EVAL), polyacrylonitrile (PAN), and others. The raw materials, manufacturers, and shapes of some of the currently available high-performance dialysis membranes are summarized in table 1. The optimal properties of dialysis membranes for efficient and safe dialysis are: high diffusion permeability, high water permeability, favorable balance between diffusion permeability and water permeability, selectivity, favorable mechanical strength when wet,

Table 1. High-performance dialysis membranes

Material	Abbreviation	Manufacturer	Membrane type
Cellulose triacetate	CTA	Nipro	hollow fiber
Polysulfone	PSf	Asahi Kasei Kuraray Medical	hollow fiber
		Fresenius	hollow fiber
		Toray	hollow fiber
Polyether sulfone	PES	Nipro	hollow fiber
		Membrana	hollow fiber
Polymethylmethacrylate	PMMA	Toray	hollow fiber
Polyester polymer alloy	PEPA	Nikkiso	hollow fiber
Ethylene vinyl alcohol copolymer	EVAL	Asahi Kasei Kuraray Medical	hollow fiber
Polyacrylonitrile	PAN	Gambro	hollow fiber laminated

biocompatibility, resistance to denaturation of the membrane material by sterilization, and cost-effectiveness [6].

Homogeneous membranes of plant-derived polymer, such as regenerated cellulose or cellulose acetate, have been used for the manufacture of dialysis membranes. Recently, asymmetrically structured dialysis membranes have been mainly used, for example synthetic polymers with high solute removal efficiency, such as PSf. Asymmetrically structured membranes are thicker than homogeneous membranes, and both the structure of the skin layer and that of the supporting layer have a significant influence on the solute permeability. A thin dense layer containing smaller pores separates solutes, while the structurally loose supporting layer provides mechanical strength and allows reinforced separation of solutes. Owing to such a skillfully designed structure, asymmetrically structured membranes remove pathogenic substances with molecular weights of several tens of thousands, which are smaller than albumin, rapidly [7].

Analysis of the Membrane Structure

The structures of membranes have been analyzed, for example by differential scanning calorimetry, calculation of pore size distribution by the nitrogen gas adsorption or dyeing method, and observation of the surface structure by electron microscopy, including scanning electron microscopy and transmission electron microscopy. However, these measurements and observation methods require pretreatments such as drying, metal sputtering, alcohol substitution and resin deposition, which may result in modification of the shape of the surface structure and of the pore structure, making analysis of the native membrane structure difficult. Examination of the pores in dialysis membranes can also be made by field-emission scanning electron microscopy; however, since metal coating is needed as a pretreatment, it is not possible to accurately determine the pore diameter. Thus, a method(s) for evaluating the pore structure at the nanometer level in wet samples, akin to clinical samples, is desired.

Atomic force microscopy (AFM) has been used in medical devices and also in the analysis of the surface properties of industrial materials since the late 1990s. AFM, which does not require pretreatment, e.g., by metal coating, provides resolution in a nanometer scale and also information on the porosity of the membrane surface and on the power spectrum density as it allows three-dimensional observation. While the presence of pores on the surface of micro-, ultra- and nanofiltration membranes can be confirmed by non-contact/tapping mode AFM, in the case of a hollow-fiber-type hemodialysis membrane with an internal diameter of approximately 200 μm, the mild waviness on the surface prevents microscopic observation by AFM [8].

Hayama et al. [8] conducted intensive studies of the method of observation of dialysis membranes by AFM, and optimized the sample fixation method, the apparatus, and the operational conditions. They examined the surface of a dialysis membrane under optimal conditions and discussed the following five items: (1) the differences in pore structure between the dry and wet states of the membrane, (2) the influence of glycerol on the pore structure and AFM images, (3) the differences in the pore structure between the internal and external surfaces, (4) the influence of a hydrophilizing agent on the pore structure, and (5) the relationship between the pore structure and the purified water filtration coefficient. They concluded from the results that AFM by the nano-microscopic method allows observation and quantitative analysis of the surface shape and the pore structure of dialysis membranes in both wet and dry states. This is the first time that clear AFM images of surface pores of a hollow-fiber dialysis membrane at such high resolution have been presented.

Yamazaki et al. [9] compared the surface structure factor of a wet membrane as determined by AFM, with the structure factor of a wet membrane calculated using the pore diffusion model, and specified the internal structure of a wet CTA membrane, which has been considered until now to be a homogeneous membrane. The AFM measurements revealed the presence of differences in the pore size between the internal and external surfaces of the wet membrane. The number of pores on the internal surface was smaller than that on the external surface, and pores branching from the internal surface to the external surface were observed. The finding that the pore size calculated using the pore diffusion model was larger than the average pore sizes of the internal and external surfaces indicated that the average pore size of the pores within the membrane was greater than that of the pores on the membrane surfaces. In addition, the membrane surface porosity, AK, of wet membranes, as determined by AFM, was smaller than the void rate H, indicating that the porosity of the internal membrane was larger than that of both surfaces. The results agree well with the concept of tortuosity in the tortuous pore diffusion model [6]. The CTA dialysis membrane, which has been considered to have a homogeneous structure, has a larger average pore size of the internal surface than that of the external surface, and has an asymmetric structure with a dense layer in the regions close to the internal and external surfaces. Such an asymmetric structure is essential for the superior solute removal efficiency of a high-performance dialysis membrane.

Acceleration of Internal Filtration

During dialysis treatment using a high-performance dialysis membrane containing large pores, because the water permeability of the membrane is very high, forward filtration of solution moving from the blood to the dialysis fluid at the blood-side inlet and also backward filtration of solution moving from the dialysis fluid to the blood at the blood-side outlet are observed [10–13]. A high-performance dialyzer with accelerated internal filtration was therefore developed, aimed at high efficient removal of high-molecular-weight substances [14]. For acceleration of internal filtration, the channel pressure drop in the dialysis fluid and/or the blood side of the dialyzer needs to be increased. The channel pressure drop in the dialyzer, ΔP, is calculated according to the following Hagen-Poiseuille equation:

$$\Delta P = \frac{128\mu LQ}{\pi d^4} \quad (1)$$

where d is the internal diameter of the channel, L is the effective length of the channel, μ is the viscosity of the fluid, and Q is the flow rate of the fluid. Equation 1 shows that when the blood flow rate and dialysis fluid flow rate are kept constant, the pressure drop increases when the channel diameter is reduced or the channel effective length is increased. Thus, dialyzers were developed in which the internal filtration can be accelerated by reduction of the internal diameter of the hollow fiber, increase in the filling rate of the hollow fiber, or increase of the effective length of the hollow fiber. For further refinement of the internal filtration-accelerated dialyzer, development of a fouling-resistant dialyzer is required by accurate evaluation of the filtration distribution inside the dialyzer. However, even if such a membrane is developed, fouling of the membrane to some extent is inevitable when filtration is initiated. Sato et al. [15] measured the flow in dialyzers by the ultrasonic Doppler method and estimated the amount of internal filtration. Development of more favorable internal filtration-accelerated dialyzers is expected using the advanced technology.

Optimization of the Dialysis Fluid Flow
Because low-molecular-weight pathogenic substances are removed by diffusion during dialysis, the flow conditions of blood and dialysis fluid in the dialyzer have a significant influence on the dialysis efficiency. In the event of channeling or obstruction (stagnation) occurring in the flow channels of blood and/or dialysis fluid, the differences in the concentrations, which are the driving force of diffusion, decrease, leading to deterioration of the dialysis efficiency. It is possible to obtain high dialysis efficiency if a uniform flow can be maintained. Even for a high-performance dialysis membrane, if the design of the dialyzer into which hollow fiber are filled is imperfect, it is not possible to obtain high performance of the dialysis membrane. Knowledge of chemical engineering would be effective for resolving this problem [6]. Factors influencing the flow in the dialyzer include the jacket shape, the hollow-fiber filling rate, and the hollow-fiber shape. In particular, the shape of the jacket varies widely among manufacturers, and various modifications of the shape are possible. An example of such modification of the jacket shape is shown in figure 1. Hirano et al. [16] discussed the influence of the jacket shape and of the hollow-fiber shape on the flow and dialysis efficiency using four kinds of dialyzer with different jacket shapes and hollow-fiber shapes, by examining the flow on the blood and dialysis fluid sides of the dialyzers by the pulse response method and measuring the clearance rates of urea, creatinine, vitamin B_{12}, and lysozyme. They concluded that the use of a full-circumference baffle and waving hollow fiber of a smaller internal diameter is effective for improvement of the dialysis efficiency; also, it is necessary to optimize the area of the slit, if the slit is formed on the long taper.

Removal of Solutes by Adsorption
PMMA dialysis membranes can remove high-molecular-weight pathogenic substances that cannot be removed by other dialysis membranes, such as cytokines and proteins, by adsorption [17, 18]. However, the precise adsorption mechanism remains unknown and needs to be elucidated, for potentially achieving more efficient removal of these pathogenic substances. The PMMA membranes used for hemodialysis have a stereocomplex structure, and it has been suggested that this peculiar structure may be involved in the adsorption of pathogenic substances with this type of membrane [19].

Biocompatibility

Prevention of Invasion of Endotoxins Contained in the Dialysis Fluid into Blood
Endotoxins (Ets) are components of the outer membranes of Gram-negative bacteria, which are released upon death of these bacteria. Ets are toxic to the body and acute symptoms such as endotoxic shock and also dialysis-related complications may occur if the Ets contained in the dialysis fluid are moved into

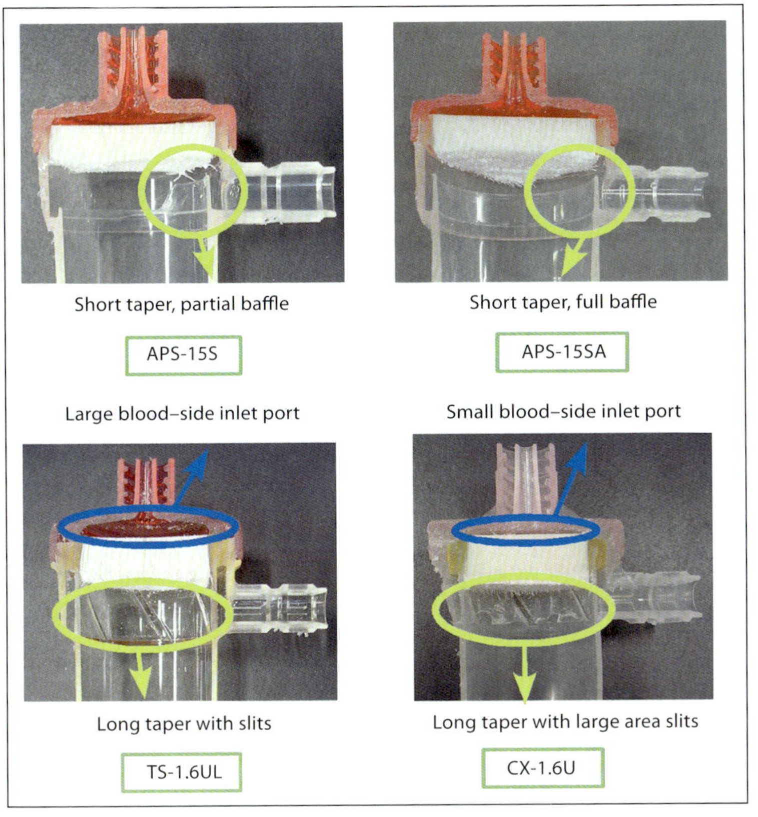

Fig. 1. Examples of modification of the jacket shape (APS-15S and APS-15SA are manufactured by Asahi Kasei Kuraray Medical, and TS-1.6UL and CX-1.6U by Toray) [16].

the blood during treatment. When a high-performance dialysis membrane is used, removal of high-molecular-weight pathogenic substances is accelerated by expansion of the pore size of the membrane and increase of filtration associated therewith, as described above, which would, however, also be associated at the same time with an increased risk of the Ets contained in the dialysis fluid moving into the patient's body by backward filtration [10–13, 20].

Hayama et al. [21] discussed the Et-trapping sites of a CTA membrane having a homogeneous structure, a PSf membrane with an internal dense layer in its structure, and a PEPA membrane having dense layers on both sides, by performing the total filtration (outside to inside) of a fluorescence-labeled Et solution. Analysis by confocal laser scanning fluorescence microscopy showed that the Ets are trapped by the outer dense layer in the case of the hydrophobic PEPA membrane, which has a dense layer on both sides; while the Ets are mostly trapped by the outer dense layer, slight trapping of Ets are also observed by the internal dense layer of the internally hydrophilized PEPA membrane. The results indicate that clogging of the membrane might contribute more to the trapped entry of the Ets into the body than the hydrophobicity of the membrane material.

Although dialysis membranes that are currently available commercially have Et-trapping capability, symptoms possibly caused by Ets, such as dialysis-related amyloidosis, are often found in patients during long-term dialysis treatment. This finding suggests that even if the Ets in the dialysis fluid do not gain entry into the blood, the Ets trapped by the dialysis membrane may interact with the blood, causing toxic symptoms during chronic treatment. Yamamoto et al. [22] developed a test method for examining the activity to the blood of the Ets trapped by hollow-fiber dialysis membranes of differing structures by backward filtration during dialysis. Currently available Et activity test methods may be used for evaluation of the activity of Ets present in solution; however, a new test method is used to measure the activity of the Ets trapped on the asymmetric dialysis membrane, involving filling of the lumen of the dialysis membrane hollow fiber with *Limulus polyphemus* corpuscular component extract. Because the pores on the internal and external surfaces of the membrane are small in diameter in the PEPA membrane, Ets are trapped mainly by the outer dense layer, and irrespective of the Et concentration of the test solution or the filtration flux, no entry of Ets into the blood or Et activity to the hollow-fiber lumen were detected. The diameter of the pores on the external surface of a PSf dialysis membrane is very large and the Ets are trapped by the internal dense layer of the hollow fiber; the Ets trapped there show activity to the hollow-fiber lumen. For suppression of Et activity during dialysis treatment, it is important to block entry of Ets into the blood and also separate the Et-trapping site from the blood.

Antioxidant Actions of Dialysis Membranes

It is known that reactive oxygen species such as superoxide and nitrogen monoxide are generated in the blood of dialysis patients, following contact with the dialysis circuit and dialysis membrane or by non-physiological flow of the blood during dialysis treatment. The reactive oxygen species increase the oxidative stress, therefore one of the important prerequisites of a dialysis membrane is that it does not generate reactive oxygen species or has the ability to remove them. Among commercially available dialysis membranes at present, a vitamin E-coated dialysis membrane has antioxidant actions and its effect in reducing the oxidative stress has been clinically confirmed [23].

Properties of the Internal Surface of a Hollow-Fiber Dialysis Membrane

Adsorption of protein on to the dialysis membrane surface triggers biological reactions, such as enhanced immune reactions. Because blood proteins are at a nanometer level in size, the properties of the dialysis membrane surface at the nanometer level exert an influence on the biocompatibility. AFM permits in-liquid observation, measurement of the surface roughness, surface softness, and also measurement of small forces such as the adsorption force between a probe-immobilized protein and a biological material surface (mapping of adsorption forces); thus, biocompatibility evaluation is also possible by nano-microscopic technology [24].

Hayama et al. [25] conducted AFM observation of the surface structure of PSf membranes differing in the PVP blending rate and molecular weight, both in the dry and wet states. The activity of lactate dehydrogenase and the amount of protein absorbed were used as indicators of the biocompatibility. They discussed the mechanism underlying the improvement of biocompatibility by blending of PVP to the PSf membrane, based on the relationship between the observed results and the biocompatibility. As a result, they concluded that the conditions favorable for improved biocompatibility are: a smaller difference in the surface roughness and a larger ratio of the diameter of the PVP particles between the wet and dry states, and higher order of alignment of the PVP particles in the wet state. Thus, the improvement of biocompatibility by PVP blending is attributable to hydration and swelling, and the resulting softening of the PVP particles on the membrane surface.

Namekawa et al. [26] examined the correlation between the internal surface properties of PEPA, EVAL and PSf dialysis membranes and the adsorption force of human serum albumin (HSA). With regard to evaluation of the properties of the internal surface of the dialysis membranes, the smoothness was determined by AFM and the percentage of PVP present on the internal surface of the dialysis membrane was determined by FT-IR. Comparison of a PEPA membrane containing no PVP with a PEPA membrane containing PVP revealed a smaller HSA-adsorbing force of the latter. Thus, containing of PVP, a hydrophilizing agent, is effective for inhibition of protein adsorption on to the dialysis membrane. A smaller HSA adsorption force was also noted for the EVAL membrane, although this membrane contains no PVP; this is attributable to the higher water content of the EVAL membrane. In addition, a positive correlation was noted between the smoothness of the PSf membrane and the HSA adsorption force ($R^2 = 0.65$). The results indicate that improvement of the smoothness of the PSf membrane is effective for inhibition of protein adsorption on to the dialysis membrane.

Koga et al. [27] developed a method for evaluation of the distribution of PVP on the surface of the dialysis membrane at the nanometer level by the novel near-field infrared microspectrometry (NFIR). Evaluation of the PVP distribution on the surface of PEPA and PSf membranes showed that the PVP is not distributed uniformly on the surface, but in a non-uniform manner, such as regions where there is no PVP, regions where there are some, and also regions where there are much, as shown in figure 2.

The above results show that the PVP distribution on the surface of current high-performance dialysis membranes is significantly uneven, when observed at the nanometer level; therefore, it is important to optimize the amount of PVP, and the sterilization conditions to improve the uniformity of the PVP distribution on the membrane surface.

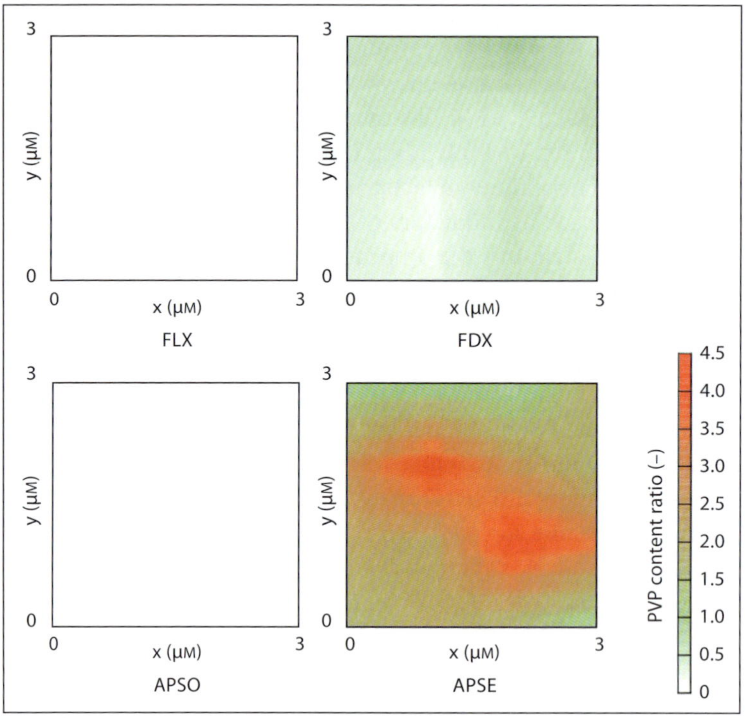

Fig. 2. PVP content ratio of dialysis membrane surface by NFIR (FLX and FDX are manufactured by Nikkiso, and APS0 and APSE by Asahi Kasei Kuraray Medical; no PVP is contained in FLX and APS0, PVP is contained in FDX and APSE) [27].

Elution of PVP

There is a concern about elution of PVP from PVP-containing synthetic polymer-based dialysis membranes, which are the mainly used high-performance dialysis membranes in clinical practice, during dialysis treatment. Elution of PVP may result in accumulation of PVP in the body and deterioration of the biocompatibility caused by the change in the surface properties of the dialysis membrane.

Namekawa et al. [28] conducted a quantitative evaluation of the PVP elution from PVP-containing dialysis membranes after different periods of storage. There is almost no risk of PVP elution from a dialysis membrane if the membrane is used immediately after sterilization; however, PVP elution becomes obvious, causing practical problems if the storage period is prolonged, particularly when the dialysis membrane is stored in a dry state. Alternatively, in the case of the PEPA membrane, which contains a smaller amount of PVP, no elution of the PVP was noted even after prolonged storage, indicating a very favorable PVP elution resistance of this membrane. The most suitable dialysis membrane for individual patients should be selected according to the storage period.

Conclusion

Most of the commercially available high-performance dialysis membranes at present are satisfactory from the point of view of the solute removal efficiency, except selectivity. However, there is still much scope for improvements in relation to the biocompatibility. Ultrahigh-performance dialysis membranes with superior biocompatibility need to be developed based on the results of basic studies carried out from the engineering point of view, reports from the manufacturers, and clinical outcomes. As further improvement in the solute removal efficiency of dialysis membranes may be difficult to expect, it may be useful to revise the current dialysis frequency of three times a week for 4 h to high-frequency dialysis or daily dialysis, and to discuss the possibility of changing the dialysis mode, in light of the possibility of home dialysis [29, 30].

References

1 Gejyo F, Yamada T, Odani S, Nakagawa Y, Arakawa M, Kunitomo T, Kataoka H, Suzuki M, Hirasawa Y, Shirahama T, Cohen A-S, Schmid K: A new form of amyloid protein associated with chronic-hemodialysis was identified as β_2-microglobulin. Biochem Biophys Res Commun 1985;129:701–706.

2 Yavuz A, Tetta C, Ersoy FF, D'Intini V, Ratanarat R, De Cal M, Bonello M, Bordoni V, Salvatori G, Andrikos E, Yakupoglu G, Levin NW, Ronco C: Uremic toxins: a new focus on an old subject. Semin Dial 2005;18: 203–211.

3 Locatelli F, Martin-Malo A, Hannedouche T, Loureiro A, Papadimitriou M, Wizemann V, Jacobson SH, Czekalski S, Ronco C, Vanholder R: Effect of membrane permeability on survival of hemodialysis patients. J Am Soc Nephrol 2009;20:645–654.

4 Gejyo F, Narita I: Current clinical and pathogenetic understanding of β_2-M amyloidosis in long-term haemodialysis patients. Nephrology 2003;8:S45–S49.

5 Bowry SK: Dialysis membranes today. Int J Artif Organs 2002;25:447–460.

6 Sakai K: Determination of pore size and pore size distribution. 2. Dialysis membranes. J Membr Sci 1994;96:91–130.

7 Yamamoto K, Hayama M, Matsuda M, Yakushiji T, Fukuda M, Miyasaka T, Sakai K: Evaluation of asymmetrical structure dialysis membrane by tortuous capillary pore diffusion model. J Membr Sci 2007;287:88–93.

8 Hayama M, Kohori F, Sakai K: AFM observation of small surface pores of hollow-fiber dialysis membrane using highly sharpened probe. J Membr Sci 2002;197: 243–249.

9 Yamazaki K, Matsuda M, Yamamoto K, Yakushiji T, Sakai K: Internal and surface structure characterization of cellulose triacetate hollow-fiber dialysis membranes. J Membr Sci 2011;368:34–40.

10 Kaneko I, Agishi T, Yamagata K, Toshihisa H, Era K, Ohta K: Technical design of hollow-fiber dialyzer (in Japanese). Jinko Zouki 1978;7:645.

11 Stiller S, Mann H, Brunner H: Backfiltration in hemodialysis with highly permeable membrane. Contrib Nephrol. Basel, Karger, 1985, vol 46, pp 23–32.

12 Hosoya N, Sakai K: Internal filtration (in Japanese). Clin Eng 1990;1:454–459.

13 Hosoya N, Kanamori T, Sakai K: Optimal design of a high-performance dialyzer involving backfiltration. Artif Organs Today 1993;2:287–298.

14 Mineshima M, Ishimori I, Ishida K, Hoshino T, Kaneko I, Sato Y, Agishi T, Tamamura N, Sakurai H, Masuda T, Hattori H: Effects of internal filtration on the solute removal efficiency of a dialyzer. ASAIO J 2000;46: 456–460.

15 Sato Y, Mineshima M, Ishimori I, Kaneko I, Akiba T, Teraoka S: Effect of hollow fiber length on solute removal and quantification of internal filtration rate by Doppler ultrasound. Int J Artif Organs 2003;26:129–134.

16 Hirano A, Yamamoto K, Matsuda M, Ogawa T, Yakushiji T, Miyasaka T, Sakai K: Evaluation of dialyzer jacket structure and hollow-fiber dialysis membranes to achieve high dialysis performance. Ther Apher Dial 2010;15:66–74.

17 Sakai K, Nagase M, Tsuda S: Adsorption of β_2-microglobulin on PMMA, PAN and cellulosic membranes. Biochem Eng J 1989;42:39–45.

18 Yamashita AC, Tomisawa N: Membrane materials for blood purification in critical care. Acute Blood Purif 2010;166:112–118.

19 Kumaki J, Kawauchi T, Okoshi K, Kusanagi H, Yashima E: Supramolecular helical structure of the stereocomplex composed of complementary isotactic and syndiotactic poly(methylmethacrylate)s as revealed by atomic force microscopy. Angew Chem Int Ed Engl 2007;46:5348–5351.

20 Hoenich NA, Levin R, Ronco C: How do changes in water quality and dialysate composition affect clinical outcomes? Blood Purif 2009;27:11–15.

21 Hayama M, Miyasaka T, Mochizuki S, Asahara H, Yamamoto K, Kohori F, Tsujioka K, Sakai K: Optimum dialysis membrane for endotoxin blocking. J Membr Sci 2003;219: 15–25.

22 Yamamoto K, Matsuda M, Hayama M, Asutagawa J, Tanaka S, Kohori F, Sakai K: Evaluation of the activity of endotoxin trapped by a hollow-fiber dialysis membrane. J Membr Sci 2006;272:211–216.

23 Cruz DN, de Cal M, Ronco C: Oxidative stress and anemia in chronic hemodialysis: the promise of bioreactive membranes. Hemodialysis: from basic research to clinical trials. Basel, Karger, 2008, vol 161, pp 89–98.

24 Mitsui K, Arakawa H, Ikai A, Nakajima K, Hara M: Dynamic measurement of single protein's mechanical properties. Biochem Biophys Res Commun 2000;272:55–63.

25 Hayama M, Yamamoto K, Kohori F, Sakai K: How polysulfone dialysis membranes containing polyvinylpyrrolidone achieve excellent biocompatibility? J Membr Sci 2004;234: 41–49.

26 Namekawa K, Fukuda M, Matsuda M, Yagi Y, Yamamoto K, Sakai K: Nanotechnological characterization of human serum albumin adsorption on wet synthetic polymer dialysis membrane surfaces. ASAIO J 2009;55: 236–242.

27 Koga S, Yakushiji T, Matsuda M, Yamamoto K, Sakai K: Functional-group analysis of polyvinylpyrrolidone on the inner surface of hollow-fiber dialysis membranes, by near-field infrared microspectroscopy. J Membr Sci 2010;355:208–213.

28 Namekawa K, Kaneko A, Sakai K, Kunikata S, Matsuda M: Longer storage of dialyzers increases elution of poly(N-vinyl-2-pyrrolidone) from polysulfone-group dialysis membranes. J Artif Organs 2011;14:52–57.

29 Kanamori T, Sakai K: Utility of short-time and frequent hemodialysis treatments from engineering points of view (in Japanese). Jinko Zouki 1991;20:1411–1420.

30 Yamashita AC, Kawanishi H: Kinetics and dose of daily hemofiltration. Blood Purif 2004;22:14–19.

Kiyotaka Sakai,
Department of Chemical Engineering, Waseda University
3-4-1 Okubo, Shinjuku-ku, Tokyo 169-8555 (Japan)
Tel. +81 3 5286 3216
E-Mail kisakai@waseda.jp

Saito A, Kawanishi H, Yamashita AC, Mineshima M (eds): High-Performance Membrane Dialyzers.
Contrib Nephrol. Basel, Karger, 2011, vol 173, pp 23–29

Biocompatible Characteristics of High-Performance Membranes

Susumu Uda[a] · Masahide Mizobuchi[b] · Tadao Akizawa[b]

[a]Division of Nephrology, Kanto Rosai Hospital, Kawasaki, and [b]Division of Nephrology, Department of Medicine, Showa University of School of Medicine, Yokohama, Japan

Abstract

Interactions of blood with hemodialysis membranes induce activation of blood factors that may cause adverse clinical outcomes in hemodialysis patients. The biocompatibility of a hemodialysis membrane is determined by the change in blood factors induced by blood interactions, and it is important that these interactions are mild and well tolerated by dialysis patients. Bioincompatible membranes that activate the complement system and accelerate cytokine production by monocytes may lead to chronic inflammation, dialysis-related amyloidosis, malnutrition, and atherosclerosis. Contact activation by a bioincompatible membrane may also induce an anaphylactoid reaction via bradykinin production. Thus, high-performance membranes should have both the high permeability to uremic substances shown by the glomerular basement membrane and the good biocompatibility of glomerular endothelial cells.

Renal replacement therapy is continuously being modified and improved. This is particularly true in hemodialysis for patients suffering from end-stage renal disease, and improvement of the characteristics of dialysis membranes is very important for a better outcome in these patients. Contact of blood with dialysis membranes and other artificial devices is unavoidable in hemodialysis and induces inflammatory responses due to activation of the immune system for recognition of 'non-self'. This causes complications in long-term dialysis therapy and may lead to adverse clinical sequelae in chronic hemodialysis patients. Thus, membrane biocompatibility and performance are important factors in the well-being and outcome of hemodialysis patients [1].

High-Performance Membranes

High-performance membranes (HPMs) have the dual properties of permeability similar to that of the glomerular basement membrane for uremic substances of small to large molecular weight (about that of albumin) and the biocompatibility of glomerular endothelial cells. Biocompatibility depends on the membrane having few interactions with blood factors. Materials with fewer interactions with blood show less activation of humoral and immunological pathways, that is, membranes that have mild effects and are well tolerated by patients are considered to be 'biocompatible' [1]. Biocompatible dialysis membranes often contain reduced or modified cellulose components and synthetic polymers, and these membranes are viewed as HPMs. Among cellulose membranes, the cellulose triacetate (CTA) membrane has been classified as a HPM.

Regenerated cellulose membranes are obtained by chemical bounding of a material to the free hydroxyl groups. However, hydroxyl groups on the surface of these membranes promote major activation of the complement system, and thus regenerated cellulose membranes are excluded from the definition of biocompatible membrane. Cellulose acetate is a modified cellulose membrane in which 80% of the hydroxyl groups of regenerated cellulose are replaced by an acetate. This suppresses complement activation, but the modification fails to prevent activation completely.

Synthetic membranes generally have higher permeability and better biocompatibility than cellulose membranes. Synthetic polymers are categorized as hydrophilic or hydrophobic and by mixing these polymers it is possible to produce a dialysis membrane with a wide flux range from low to high. Membrane biocompatibility is determined by a low energy of interaction with water, protein adsorption, size and distribution of pores, and a high ultrafiltration coefficient. Hydrophobic membranes generally have these characteristics, but need to be rendered hydrophilic by addition of a polymer such as polyvinylpyrrolidone (PVP). Hydrophobic membranes in common use include those made from polysulfone (PS), polymethylmethacrylate (PMMA), polyamide (PA), polyacrylonitrile (PAN), polyethersulfone (PES), and polyesterpolymeralloy (PEPA) while hydrophilic membranes include those based on polyethylene-co-vinyl alcohol (EVAL) (table 1).

HPMs should be biocompatible and should also be able to remove target substances efficiently. Thus, HPMs should have high capacity for removal of protein-bound or large-molecular-weight substances, including β_2-microglobulin, a major pathogen in dialysis-related amyloidosis, and uremic toxins that are larger than albumin. Moreover, the membrane should have a high-molecular-weight cut-off, a sharp cut-off curve, and greater adsorption capacity [1].

Table 1. Hydrophobic membranes in common use

Membrane type	Membrane character
Cellulosic	
Cellulose	
Modified cellulosic	
Cellulose diacetate	Hydroxyl groups replaced with acetate
Cellulose triacetate (CTA)	Hydroxyl groups replaced with acetate
Hemophane	Hydroxyl groups replaced with diethylaminoethyl redicals
Synthetic polymers	
Ethylvinyl alcohol (EVAL)	Hydrophilic
Polysulfone (PS)	Hydrophobic
Polymethylmethacrylate (PMMA)	Hydrophobic
Polyacrylonitrile (PAN)	Hydrophobic
Polyamide (PA)	Hydrophobic
Polyethersulfone (PES)	Hydrophobic
Polyesterpolymeralloy (PEPA)	Hydrophobic

Typical types of hemodialysis membranes.

Complement and Neutrophil Activation

Creddock et al. [2] first demonstrated that dialysis-induced leukopenia is caused by activation of complement during hemodialysis using cellulose membranes. This activation reaches a maximum at 15 min after the start of dialysis and lasts for up to 90 min [3]. Complement activation occurs via the alternate pathway during hemodialysis and leads to neutrophil activation and subsequently to sequestration of neutrophils in pulmonary vessels and the circulation. Products of this activation, including C3b and C5a (anaphylatoxins), are released and result in vascular smooth muscle contraction, increased vascular permeability, and inflammation. Use of a PAN membrane minimizes complement activation and does not induce leukopenia [4]. In contrast, a PS membrane can activate the complement system, but the products of activation are fully adsorbed by the membrane.

Contact Pathway Activation

Contact pathway activation occurs after blood contact with the membrane surface, especially if this surface is negatively charged. This pathway is initiated by factor XII (Hageman factor) activation. A high incidence of anaphylactoid reactions is observed in cases with hemodialysis using a PAN (AN69) membrane (which has a negative surface charge) and concomitant use of angiotensin-converting enzyme (ACE) inhibitors. The final product of the contact pathway, bradykinin, induces the anaphylactoid reaction [5]. However, enhanced bradykinin production is often well tolerated because it is rapidly inactivated by kininase II. Since ACE is also a kininase II [6], the likelihood of an anaphylactoid reaction is increased when patients undergoing hemodialysis are also taking ACE inhibitors [7, 8].

Platelet-Neutrophil Interactions

Platelet-neutrophil microaggregates are observed in the blood in the early phase of hemodialysis [9]. Formation of the microaggregates is mediated by an interaction between P-selectin expressed on the surface of activated platelets due to blood-membrane contacts and P-selectin glycoprotein ligand-1 on the neutrophil surface. P-selectin-mediated adhesion of activated platelets to neutrophils increases the production of reactive oxygen species [10, 11] and tumor necrosis factor-α. This phenomenon suggests that repetitive hemodialysis per se may cause an inflammatory state in chronic hemodialysis patients.

Recovery from Acute Kidney Injury

The type of hemodialysis membrane that promotes survival and recovery from acute kidney injury remains a controversial issue, since several prospective randomized trials have shown significantly higher survival and renal recovery rates after hemodialysis with a biocompatible membrane compared to a bioincompatible membrane [12–14], whereas other studies have not shown this difference [15–18].

Chronic Outcomes of Bioincompatibility

Henderson et al. proposed the interleukin hypothesis that dialysis-induced cytokine production leads to complications in dialysis patients. Pro-inflammatory cytokines are produced via activation of mononuclear cells due to complement activation on the cellulose membrane, and endotoxins, fragments of endotoxins, and acetate in the dialysate may be transferred from the dialysate to the blood. This hypothesis was initially applied to acute complications of hemodialysis therapy such as dialysis hypotension. However, it is now used for a broader interpretation of chronic complications of dialysis patients, including chronic inflammation, dialysis-related amyloidosis, malnutrition inflammation, and atherosclerosis (MIA) syndrome [19].

Thus, membranes with a greater pore size, reduced thickness, and lower adsorptive capacity for endotoxin, which are representative characteristics of bioincompatible membranes, permit greater passage of substances from contaminated dialysate that induce tumor necrosis factor-α production by monocytes [20].

Several reports have shown that hemodialysis using biocompatible membranes is associated with lower morbidity and mortality compared to hemodialysis with bioincompatible membranes. For example, in the 4D study (post-hoc analysis) of four different types of membranes (high-flux synthetic, low-flux synthetic, low-flux semisynthetic (cellulose acetate), and low-flux cellulose), a significantly greater risk of death was found in patients treated with low-flux cellulose and low-flux semisynthetic membranes compared with low-flux synthetic membranes [21].

In dialysis-related amyloidosis, β_2-microglobulin (MW 11,800) is the major amyloid fibril component. Dialysis-related amyloidosis has a harmful influence on the QOL of long-term hemodialysis patients. There is some evidence that the use of biocompatible membranes contributes to delaying the onset of dialysis-related amyloidosis. Koda et al. [22] showed that the incidence of carpal tunnel syndrome was lower and that survival was improved in patients treated with a biocompatible membrane compared to those treated with a bioincompatible membrane.

The hemodialysis membrane also plays an important role in susceptibility to infection [23]. Changing the membrane from bioincompatible to biocompatible decreases the incidence of infection among causes of death and in hospitalization [24], since chronic hemodialysis with a bioincompatible membrane leads to attenuation of metabolic responses to phagocytic stimuli to a greater extent than that with a biocompatible membrane. Malnutrition also often occurs in hemodialysis patients and is related to increased mortality. An acceleration of catabolism is evident on hemodialysis days and it has been suggested that the malnutritional status is associated with the bioincompatibility of the hemodialysis membrane [25, 26].

Conclusion

Hemodialysis is a repetitive process that is performed over a long period, which indicates that even low-grade or minor membrane-related adverse reactions need to be avoided. Therefore, HPMs should be used that produce weak inflammatory stimuli due to good biocompatibility and have a high capacity for removal of uremic substances with minimum loss of essential substances for the body.

References

1 Akizawa T, Kinugasa E, Koiwa F, Kohjiro S, Ideura T: Dialysis membranes in the year 2000: Performance and biocompatibility. Nephrol Dial Transplant 1996;11(suppl 8): 16–19.

2 Craddock PR, Fehr J, Dalmasso AP, Brighan KL, Jacob HS: Hemodialysis leukopenia. Pulmonary vascular leukostasis resulting from complement activation by dialyzer cellophane membranes. J Clin Invest 1977;59: 879–888.

3 Hakim RM: Clinical implications of hemodialysis membrane biocompatibility. Kidney Int 1993;44:484–494.

4 Chenoweth DE, Cheung AK, Henderson LW: Anaphylatoxin formation during hemodialysis: effects of different dialyzer membranes. Kidney Int 1983;24:764–769.

5 Verresen L, Fink E, Lemke HD, Vanrenterghem Y: Bradykinin is a mediator of anaphylactoid reactions during hemodialysis with AN69 membranes. Kidney Int 1994;45:1497–1503.

6 Zusman RM: Renin- and non-renin-mediated antihypertensive actions of converting enzyme inhibitors. Kidney Int 1984; 25:969–983.

7 Tielemans C, Madhoun P, Lenaers M, Schandene L, Goldman M, Vanherweghem JL: Anaphylactoid reactions during hemodialysis on AN69 membranes in patients receiving ACE inhibitors. Kidney Int 1990; 38:982–984.

8 Parnes EL, Shapiro WB: Anaphylactoid reactions in hemodialysis patients treated with the AN69 dialyzer. Kidney Int 1991;40:1148–1152.

9 Gawaz MP, Mujais SK, Schmidt B, Gurland HJ: Platelet-leukocyte aggregation during hemodialysis. Kidney Int 1994;46:489–495.

10 Bonomini M, Stuard S, Carreno MP, Settefrati N, Santarelli P, Haeffner-Cavaillon N, Albertazzi A: Neutrophil reactive oxygen species production during hemodialysis: role of activated platelet adhesion to neutrophils through P-selectin. Nephron 1997;75:402–411.

11 Nagata K, Tsuji T, Todoroki N, Katagiri Y, Tanoue K, Yamazaki H, Hanai N, Irimura T: Activated platelets induce superoxide anion release by monocytes and neutrophils through P-selectin (CD62). J Immunol 1993; 151:3267–3273.

12 Hakim RM, Wingard RL, Parker RA: Effect of the dialysis membrane in the treatment of patients with acute renal failure. N Engl J Med 1994;331:1338–1342.

13 Schiffl H, Lang SM, Konig A, Strasser T, Haider MC, Held E: Biocompatible membranes in acute renal failure: prospective case-controlled study. Lancet 1994;344: 570–572.

14 Himmelfarb J, Tolkoff Rubin N, Chandran P, Parker RA, Wingard RL, Hakim R: A multicenter comparison of dialysis membranes in the treatment of acute renal failure requiring dialysis. J Am Soc Nephrol 1998;9:257–266.

15 Jorres A, Gahl GM, Dobis C, Polenakovic MH, Cakalaroski K, Rutkowski B, Kisielnicka E, Krieter DH, Rumpf KW, Guenther C, Gaus W, Hoegel J: Haemodialysis-membrane biocompatibility and mortality of patients with dialysis-dependent acute renal failure: a prospective randomised multicentre trial. International multicentre study group. Lancet 1999;354:1337–1341.

16 Gastaldello K, Melot C, Kahn RJ, Vanherweghem JL, Vincent JL, Tielemans C: Comparison of cellulose diacetate and polysulfone membranes in the outcome of acute renal failure. A prospective randomized study. Nephrol Dial Transplant 2000;15: 224–230.

17 Alonso A, Lau J, Jaber BL: Biocompatible hemodialysis membranes for acute renal failure. Cochrane Database Syst Rev 2005:CD005283.

18 Vanholder R, Lameire N: Does biocompatibility of dialysis membranes affect recovery of renal function and survival? Lancet 1999;354:1316–1318.

19 Stenvinkel P, Heimburger O, Paultre F, Diczfalusy U, Wang T, Berglund L, Jogestrand T: Strong association between malnutrition, inflammation, and atherosclerosis in chronic renal failure. Kidney Int 1999;55:1899–1911.

20 Lonnemann G, Koch KM, Shaldon S, Dinarello CA: Studies on the ability of hemodialysis membranes to induce, bind, and clear human interleukin-1. J Lab Clin Med 1988;112:76–86.

21 Krane V, Krieter DH, Olschewski M, Marz W, Mann JF, Ritz E, Wanner C: Dialyzer membrane characteristics and outcome of patients with type 2 diabetes on maintenance hemodialysis. Am J Kidney Dis 2007;49: 267–275.
22 Koda Y, Nishi S, Miyazaki S, Haginoshita S, Sakurabayashi T, Suzuki M, Sakai S, Yuasa Y, Hirasawa Y, Nishi T: Switch from conventional to high-flux membrane reduces the risk of carpal tunnel syndrome and mortality of hemodialysis patients. Kidney Int 1997;52: 1096–1101.
23 Vanholder R, Ringoir S: Infectious morbidity and defects of phagocytic function in end-stage renal disease: a review. J Am Soc Nephrol 1993;3:1541–1554.
24 Hornberger JC, Chernew M, Petersen J, Garber AM: A multivariate analysis of mortality and hospital admissions with high-flux dialysis. J Am Soc Nephrol 1992;3: 1227–1237.
25 Gutierrez A, Alvestrand A, Wahren J, Bergstrom J: Effect of in vivo contact between blood and dialysis membranes on protein catabolism in humans. Kidney Int 1990;38:487–494.
26 Gutierrez A, Alvestrand A, Bergstrom J: Membrane selection and muscle protein catabolism. Kidney Int Suppl 1992;38: S86–90.

Susumu Uda
Division of Nephrology, Kanto Rosai Hospital
Kizukisumiyoshi-cho, Nakahara-ku
Kawasaki, Kanagawa 221-8510 (Japan)
Tel. +81 44 411 3131, E-Mail suda@kantoh.rofuku.go.jp

Saito A, Kawanishi H, Yamashita AC, Mineshima M (eds): High-Performance Membrane Dialyzers.
Contrib Nephrol. Basel, Karger, 2011, vol 173, pp 30–35

Selection Guidelines for High-Performance Membrane

Tsutomu Sanaka[a] · Masahide Koremoto[b]

[a]Division of Nephrology and Blood Purification, Tokyo Women's Medical University Medical Center East, Tokyo, and [b]Scientific and Technical Affairs Department, Dialysis Products Division, Asahikasei Kuraray Medical Co., Ltd, Tokyo, Japan

Abstract

The fundamental concept for the selection of high-performance membrane is based on solute removal capability and biocompatibility. From this principle, the selection guidelines for high-performance membrane are recommended as follows: (1) The currently available products do not provide coverage of the necessary 'balance between solute removal and biocompatibility' in a single dialyzer for all the dialysis patients. Therefore, it is advisable to choose a high-performance membrane taking into consideration the balance between the solute removal capacity necessary for the patient and the severity of complications that is considered a surrogate marker for biocompatibility. (2) There is an increasing demand in dialysis therapy for new biocompatibility indices such as 'reducing blood pressure variability during dialysis', 'decreasing oxidative stress' and 'delaying the onset or progression of complications'. High-performance membranes developed to address these needs include the ethylene-co-vinyl alcohol copolymer (EVAL) (R) membrane, cellulose triacetate, polymethylmethacrylate, vitamin E-coated polysulfone (PS) membrane, and PS membrane hemodiafiltration filter.

Aiming at further improvement of the survival outcome of patients on chronic dialysis, dialyzers have been continuously developed from the viewpoints of (1) improving the removal capability of uremic substances, (2) improving biocompatibility, (3) combining glomerular function and renal tubular function. As a result, various high-performance membranes are now available commercially.

On the other hand, the disease states of patients on chronic dialysis vary depending on the history of dialysis, age, underlying disease, and complications. At the same time, the degree of accumulation of uremic substances in the body also differs among individual patients. Obviously, it is necessary to choose a dialyzer that is compatible with the disease state of individual patient.

This article summarizes the concepts that should form the selection criteria of high-performance membrane, based on a comprehensive review of the literature.

Fundamental Concepts Related to Choice of High-Performance Membrane

Solute Removal Capability

First and foremost, the selection of high-performance membrane should consider the properties of removal and leakage of uremic substances that range from small molecular substances represented by urea, creatinine, uric acid and inorganic phosphate, to protein molecules with sizes from β_2-microglobulin (MG) to albumin. For the removal of solutes ranging from small molecular substances to β_2-MG, the present technological development of polysulfone (PS) membrane has reached a level that has been considered to be the target performance. Therefore, selection of membranes with this level of capability is now possible.

For solute removal up to the level of albumin, dialyzers are required to possess the function of removal uremic toxins by albumin binding. In this case, it is necessary to remove a certain amount of albumin. For this purpose also, it is possible to choose from commercial products a high-performance membrane that is compatible with the clinical state, the nutrition status, and the metabolic efficiency of the dialysis patient, as well as the therapeutic policy of the physician.

Biocompatibility

As indices of general biocompatibility, changes in white blood cell count and platelet count during dialysis, activation of complement, and residual blood volume after dialysis have been reported by many clinical studies of commercial products [1–3]. According to these clinical studies, changes in white blood cell and platelet counts during dialysis, activation of complement, and residual blood after dialysis are the basic criteria. At the same time, while the issues of the kinetics of various cytokines in the body and exposure to oxidative stress should be considered, these cannot be measured in the routine clinical setting. Under such circumstances, inadequacy in biocompatibility has to be identified from the changes in clinical state as indicated by biomarkers such as response of renal anemia to erythropoietin-stimulating agent, inflammatory pathology, cardiovascular complications, arteriosclerosis, and low nutrition syndrome. Based on these assessments, an appropriate high-performance membrane has to be selected.

Fortunately, the commercially available dialysis membranes have almost achieved the target levels of biocompatibility. However, apart from the conventional biocompatibility, there is an increasing demand to consider also biocompatibility that reflects the QOL. It is a fact that new indicators of biocompatibility reflecting QOL, such as 'reducing blood pressure variability during dialysis', 'decreasing oxidative stress' and 'delaying the onset or progression of complications' have become new targets for the development of high-performance membranes.

Evaluation Reports as References for Selection of High-Performance Membrane

Solute Removal Capability

While the small molecular substances that constitute the majority of uremic substances can be removed by diffusion, solutes in the range of low-molecular-weight proteins are removed by filtration. When considering the balance between removal and leakage prevention for human β_2-MG, human α_1-MG, and human albumin, since the current technology has almost cleared the removal target for β_2-MG, the balance can be observed by plotting albumin leakage on the x-axis and α_1-MG removal rate on the y-axis. When this is examined for different membranes, the APS-E, APS-EL, and APS-EX dialyzers (Asahikasei Kuraray Medical Co., Ltd) appear to achieve a better balance among various products.

Biocompatibility

Reports on general biocompatibility as reflected by changes in white blood cell and platelet counts during dialysis, complement activation during dialysis, and residual blood volume after dialysis (indicated by the minimum heparin dosage) showed that APS-E, APS-EL, and APS-EX dialyzers have almost reached the target levels [4].

Overall Evaluation of Solute Removal and Biocompatibility

To objectively evaluate the performance of dialyzers including the balance between solute removal capability and biocompatibility, we conducted a literature search of international articles and summarized the characteristics of various dialyzers in table 1. The search was conducted using PubMed [http://www.ncbi.nlm.nih.gov/sites/entrez] using keywords that include the following: [dialysis (dialyzer or dialyser)] and (EVAL or APS or vitamin E or REXEED). The search extracted 80 articles with dialyzer as research subject as of February 26, 2009. Among these articles, 70 articles reported on the characteristics of APS series, KF series, vitamin E membrane series (table 1).

Regarding the contents of the articles judged from the characteristics of the research area, articles on vitamin E-coated dialyzers and ethylene-co-vinyl

Table 1. Review of literature on solute removal capability and biocompatibility of high-performance membrane as of February 26, 2009[1]

	Removal property	Anti-thrombotic property	Lower cellular stimulation	Improve anemia	Improve arterio-sclerosis	Lower oxidative stress	Improve indefinite compliant	Reduce inflammation	Improve hypotension
PS series	11	1	2						
EVAL series		5	1		1				
PS (vitamin E-coated)						1			
Cellulose (vitamin E-coated)	2	2	8	4	6	20	2	7	1

[1] The search was conducted using PubMed [http://www.ncbi.nlm.nih.gov/sites/entrez]. Studies on dialyzers (including overseas products): number of articles identified by key words = 80; superiority data obtained from characteristic studies = 70; overlap (including overlapping characteristics) = 4.

alcohol (EVAL) (R) membrane dialyzers were mostly associated with biocompatibility including the relation with oxidative stress. On the other hand, articles on APS series dialyzers were mainly on the removal capability, with some reporting on general biocompatibility such as residual blood volume.

Selection Guidelines for High-Performance Membrane

As the above discussions show, the currently available products do not really provide coverage of the necessary 'balance between solute removal and biocompatibility' in a single dialyzer for all the dialysis patients. Therefore, it is advisable to choose a high-performance membrane taking into consideration the balance between the solute removal capacity necessary for the patient and the severity of the complications that is considered a surrogate marker for biocompatibility (fig. 1).

Furthermore, there is an increasing demand in dialysis therapy for new biocompatibility indices such as 'reducing blood pressure variability during dialysis', 'decreasing oxidative stress' and 'delaying the onset or progression of complications'. To address these needs, high-performance membranes such as EVAL (R) membrane, vitamin E-coated PS membrane, and PS membrane hemodiafiltration filter are already being marketed. In other words, these can

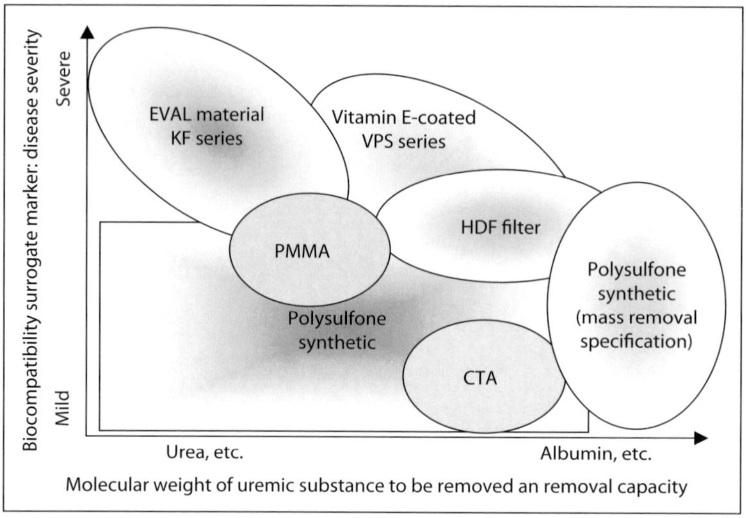

Fig. 1. Selection guideline for high-performance membrane: overall evaluation of solute removal and biocompatibility.

be regarded as products for counteracting 'dysdialysis syndrome or hypotension during dialysis' [5–9].

The number of diabetic dialysis patients is increasing every year, and these patients are prone to develop hypotension during dialysis [10–15]. With this background, a multicenter trial was conducted in diabetic dialysis patients to observe the variation in blood pressure during dialysis upon changing the conventional dialyzer to vitamin E-coated PS membrane dialyzer VPS-HA [16]. After using the VPS-HA for 3 months, a significant attenuation in systolic pressure lowering during the latter half of dialysis was observed, together with a tendency of dose reduction of presser agent. In addition, serum albumin was significant increased, showing interesting results.

Conclusion

If the concept of developing and selecting dialyzers closer to the biological kidney is to be pursued in the future, the issues including 'aging' and 'increase in diabetic dialysis patients' should be addressed. In actual fact, the survival outcome of dialysis patients is becoming poorer, in contrast to the recognition so far [17]. Physicians who are engaged in treating patients today should be aware that with the increasing sophistication of medical technology, the demand from patients for excellent biocompatibility will grow even stronger in the future [16].

References

1 Sagae O, Suzuki M, Tanata T, et al: Performance assessment of APS-U (in Japanese). Jin To Toseki (Kidney & Dialysis) 2004;57(Suppl High-Performance Membrane '04):46–50.

2 Miyawaki N, Takata S, Minami M, et al: Assessment of biocompatibility and solute removal performance of polysulfone membrane dialyzer APS-U (in Japanese). Jin To Toseki (Kidney & Dialysis) 2003;55(Suppl High-Performance Membrane '03):126–129.

3 Tsukamoto I, Murasugi H, Yamashita Y, et al: Does the difference in anticoagulant dosage obtained from residual blood assessment of different types of dialyzers indicate change in lipids during dialysis? (in Japanese) Vitamembrane 2007;7:6–12.

4 Japanese Society for Dialysis Therapy: Illustration of current status of chronic dialysis treatment in Japan, as of December 31, 2007 (in Japanese).

5 Yamamoto K, Matsunaga A, Saito M, et al: Analysis of the mechanisms underlying excessive blood pressure lowering during maintenance hemodialysis (in Japanese, Engl abstr). Nihon Toseki Igakkai Zasshi 2007;40: 897–906.

6 Inoue M, Kusano E: Blood pressure control in patients with diabetic renal insufficiency: symptoms and treatment (in Japanese). Toseki Kea (Japanese Journal of Dialysis & Caring) 2005;II(12):1230–1231.

7 Matsunaga T: Hypotension and hypertension during dialysis (in Japanese). Toseki Kea (Japanese Journal of Dialysis & Caring) 2007(Winter Suppl):42–45.

8 Hisanaga S: Prevention and treatment of cardiovascular changed during dialysis (in Japanese). Toseki Kea (Japanese Journal of Dialysis & Caring) 2006(Summer Suppl):288–295.

9 Williams B: A potential role for angiotensin II-induced vascular endothelial growth factor expression in the pathogenesis of diabetic nephropathy? Miner Electrolyte Metab 1998; 24:400–405.

10 Williamson JR, Chang K, Frangos M, et al: Hyperglycemic pseudo-hypoxia and diabetic complications. Diabetes 1993;42:801–803.

11 Miyata S, Monnier V: Immunohistochemical detection of advanced glycosylation end products in diabetic tissues using monoclonal antibody to pyrraline. J Clin Invest 1992; 89:1102–1112.

12 Nishizuka Y: Intracellular signaling by hydrolysis of phospholipids and activation of protein kinase C. Science 1992;258: 607–614.

13 King GL, Kunisaki M, Nishio Y, et al: Biochemical and molecular mechanisms in the development of diabetic vascular complications. Diabetes 1996;45(suppl 3): S105–S108.

14 Baynes JW, Thorpe SR: Role of oxidative stress in diabetic complications: a new perspective on an old paradigm. Diabetes 1999;48:1–9.

15 Thomas KA: Vascular endothelial growth factor, a potent and selective angiogenic agent. J Biol Chem 1996;271:603–606.

16 Matsumura M, Sasaki H, Sekizuka K, Sano H, Ogawa K, Shimizu C, Yoshida H, Kobayashi S, Koremoto M, Aritomi M, Ueki K: Improved management of intradialytic hypotension using vitamin E-bonded polysulfone membrane dialyzer. Int J Artif Organs 2010;33:147–153.

17 Koremoto M: Hemodialysis membrane function and membrane development accompanying aging and increase in diabetic patients: approach in the hollow-type dialysis membrane development for improving removal capability and biocompatibility (in Japanese). WEB J 2005;68:35–38.

Tsutomu Sanaka, MD, PhD
Division of Nephrology and Blood Purification
Tokyo Women's Medical University Medical Center East
2-1-10 Nishiogu, Arakawaku, Tokyo 116-8567 (Japan)
Tel. +81 3 3810 1111, E-Mail tsnkkc@dnh.twmu.ac.jp

Saito A, Kawanishi H, Yamashita AC, Mineshima M (eds): High-Performance Membrane Dialyzers.
Contrib Nephrol. Basel, Karger, 2011, vol 173, pp 36–43

Preferred Performance of the High-Performance Membrane in the Case of Online Hemodiafiltration

Hideki Kawanishi

Tsuchiya General Hospital, Hiroshima, Japan

Abstract

High-performance membrane (HPM) dialyzers have become commonly used in online hemodiafiltration (ol-HDF). HPM dialyzers with a markedly improved function of removing high-molecular solutes have appeared, but excessive albumin loss often occurs using these. Higher albumin loss was observed when these protein-permeable dialyzers were used for post-dilution ol-HDF. When albumin loss is regarded as the criterion, dialyzers with a 0.5 g or lower albumin loss in the hemodialysis mode should be used for post-dilution HDF, whereas those with a 2 g or greater albumin loss should be selected for pre-dilution HDF. The performance of recent HPM dialyzers has been markedly developed, and equivalent removal efficiency can now be achieved with non-ol-HDF. To demonstrate the efficacy of ol-HDF, it is necessary to compare hemodialysis and ol-HDF using a type V dialyzer (β_2-microglobulin clearance ≥70 ml/min) classified in Japan, and re-investigate the significance of removing high-molecular solutes larger than β_2-microglobulin and protein-bound solutes.

It is widely known that the survival rate of Japanese dialysis patients is the highest in the world [1]. This is mainly due to the development of dialysis and blood purification devices and preparation of the dialysis system and cooperation among academic societies, the clinical engineering technologists, and industries has also played a significant role. Especially, the introduction of the central dialysis fluid delivery system (CDDS) in the 1960s realized the provision of stable dialysis conditions for all patients, which made a marked contribution. This favorable survival rate has been achieved by applying standardized dialysis under identical conditions (4 h, 3 times a week using a super high-flux membrane) at all facilities nationwide.

In this dialysis environment, online hemodiafiltration (ol-HDF) has inevitably developed into central ol-HDF since the 1990s [2, 3].

High-functional dialyzers have also been developed rapidly at the same time, products termed high-performance membrane (HPM) dialyzers became clinically applicable, and these HPM dialyzers have become commonly used in ol-HDF. HPM dialyzers with a markedly improved function of removing high-molecular solutes have appeared, but excessive albumin loss often occurs using these. Higher albumin loss was observed when these protein-permeable dialyzers were used for post-dilution ol-HDF [4]. Thus, elevation of the efficiency of high-molecular solutes removal while controlling albumin loss by employing pre-dilution ol-HDF has become actively performed.

The superior efficiency of protein-bound substance removal in this pre-dilution ol-HDF, compared to that in post-dilution ol-HDF, has been pointed out [5, 6], and pre-dilution ol-HDF using a protein-permeable HPM dialyzer has become the main trend in Japan.

In this article, the removal characteristics of ol-HDF using HPM dialyzers are discussed.

Calculation of Clearance by ol-HDF

To determine clearance by ol-HDF, summing of diffusion and convection is necessary. However, the addition of diffusion makes pre-dilution HDF complex. Moreover, the dialysate flow is reduced as the convection volume is increased in ol-HDF, reducing the efficiency of diffusion.

The clearance calculation formula of ol-HDF is shown in figure 1 [7]. Changes in clearance with variation of the convective volume within a molecular weight range from urea to β_2-microglobulin (BMG) were calculated using this formula for pre- and post-dilution ol-HDF. The results are shown in figure 2. The clearance of all substances increased as the convective volume increased in post-dilution HDF.

In pre-dilution HDF, the clearance of high-molecular solutes, such as BMG and inulin, by convection was greater than that by diffusion, and the total clearance increased with convective volume, but, inversely, the total clearance of low-molecular solutes, such as urea and creatinine, decreased because the concentration flowing into the dialyzer decreased, reducing the clearance by diffusion.

Therefore, not only convection but also diffusion (mass transfer coefficient, KoA) is an important element of HDF, for which the use of a HPM is essential [8]. In Japan, HPM dialyzers have been actively employed in HDF.

$$K_O = Q_B \left[\frac{\exp\left[N_T(1-Z)\right]-1}{\exp\left[N_T(1-Z)\right]-Z} \right]$$

$$K_{HDF\ pre} = \left[K_{O\ pre} + S_C Q_F \left(1 - \frac{K_{O\ pre}}{Q_B + Q_F}\right) \right] \left(\frac{O_B}{Q_B + Q_F} \right)$$

$$K_{HDF\ post} = K_{O\ post} + S_C Q_F \left(1 - \frac{K_{O\ post}}{Q_B}\right)$$

$$K_{HDF\ pre\ \&\ post} = \left[K_{O\ pre\ \&\ post} + S_C Q_F \left(1 - \frac{K_{O\ pre\ \&\ post}}{Q_B + \text{pre}\ Q_F}\right) \right] \left(\frac{Q_B}{Q_B + \text{pre}\ Q_F} \right)$$

$$Z_{HD} = \frac{Q_B}{Q_D} \quad Z_{post} = \frac{Q_B}{Q_D} \quad Z_{pre} = \frac{Q_B + Q_F + Q_F}{Q_D} \quad Z_{pre\ \&\ post} = \frac{Q_B + \text{pre}\ Q_F}{Q_D}$$

$$N_{T\ HD} = \frac{KoA}{Q_D} \quad N_{T\ post} = \frac{KoA}{Q_D} \quad N_{T\ pre} = \frac{KoA}{Q_B + Q_F} \quad N_{T\ pre\ \&\ post} = \frac{KoA}{Q_B + \text{pre}\ Q_F}$$

Fig. 1. Simulation of solute clearance on HDF. K = Clearance; Sc = sieving coefficient; KoA = mass transfer area coefficient, Q_F = convection rate; Q_D = dialysis fluid flow; Q_B = blood flow. In ol-HDF, Q_D is changed according to Q_F.

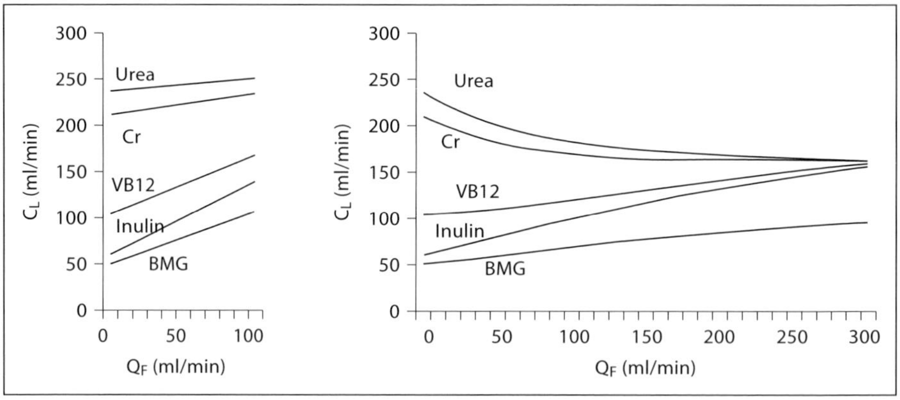

Fig. 2. Simulation of clearance of ol-HDF, left post-dilution ol-HDF, right pre-dilution ol-HDF, blood flow 300 ml/min, dialysate flow 700 ml/min, KoA of urea 600, Cr 450, VB12 140, inulin 70, and BMG 60 ml/min, sieving coefficient of urea 1.0, Cr 1.0, VB12 1.0, inulin 1.0, and BMG 0.75.

Setting of Convective Volume in ol-HDF

The bases of setting the convective volume in ol-HDF are the water permeability of the dialyzer and blood flow. Methods include setting a percentage of the blood flow (flow control) and setting by observing changes in the transmembrane pressure (TMP) (pressure control) [9]. Since the blood and protein concentrations vary among patients, it is difficult to continuously maintain the maximum convective volume in the flow control method. The pressure control method is simple and stable, in which an upper TMP limit of 300 mm Hg inevitably sets the upper limit at one third to one fourth of the blood flow for post-dilution ol-HDF and about twice the blood flow for pre-dilution ol-HDF. Since TMP changes (rises) with the course of dialysis, the convective volume is decreased with it. However, this method is employed to obtain the maximum convective volume in individual patients. To compare the clinical effect, the convective volume should be set employing a specific system.

Many large-scale studies on ol-HDF have recently been reported, but, unexpectedly, only a few studies clearly defined the convective volume. Vilar et al. [10] set the convective volume at 35% of the blood flow because it depends on the blood flow in post-dilution HDF. Santoro et al. [11] set the total convective volume at 120% of the dry weight in ol-HF. Regarding the pre-dilution procedure, Locatelli et al. [12] set the convective volume at 100% of the blood flow (60 l/session, 106% of the dry weight) in ol-HF and 60% (40 l/session, 64% of the dry weight) in ol-HDF. In Japan, as described below, pre-dilution ol-HDF using a protein-permeable dialyzer is frequently performed, and the convective volume is generally set at 100–150% of the blood flow (60–72 l/session) because the blood flow is lower (250–300 ml/min) than that in HDF in other countries.

Dialyzer Performance and Dilution Method in ol-HDF

When pre- and post-dilutions are employed, the dilution system is limited by the dialyzer used. The removal efficiency can be increased by adding as much convection as possible, but it is limited because albumin loss increases. The dialyzer and dilution method are selected based on how to separate removed high-molecular solutes from albumin loss.

Using a non-protein-permeable dialyzer for post-dilution HDF, the BMG (MW 11.7 kDa) clearance increased in proportion to the increase in the convective volume. Albumin loss was controlled, but the α_1-microglobulin (AMG, MW 33 kDa) clearance was also low. On the other hand, when it was used for pre-dilution HDF, no higher efficiency than that in post-dilution HDF was achieved, even though the convective volume was increased.

In contrast, when a protein-permeable dialyzer was used for post-dilution HDF, the BMG and AMG clearances increased, but albumin loss also rapidly increased with them. On the other hand, when it was employed for pre-dilution HDF, albumin loss was controlled, while the AMG clearance also increased.

When a dialyzer with a 2 g or more albumin loss in the hemodialysis (HD) mode per session is used for post-dilution HDF, albumin of 5 g or more is lost. When albumin loss is regarded as the criterion, dialyzers with a 0.5 g or lower albumin loss in the HD mode per session should be used for post-dilution HDF,

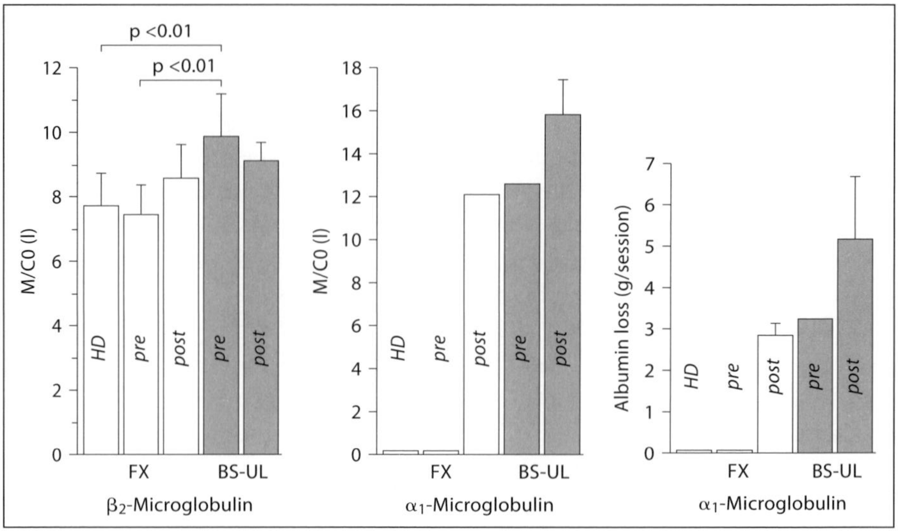

Fig. 3. Comparison of protein-permeable HPM dialyzer (BS-2.1UL) and protein-non-permeable HPM dialyzer (FX220) on the removal capacity in different dilution mode. M/CO = Removal volume per solute concentration; pre = pre-dilution, post = post-dilution, blood flow 250 ml/min, dialysate flow 500 ml/min, convective volume: pre-dilution 70 l/session, post-dilution 16 l/session, dialysis time 240 min.

whereas those with a 2 g or greater albumin loss should be selected for pre-dilution HDF.

The removal characteristics of a protein-permeable dialyzer, BS-2.1UL (Toray Medical, Co. Ltd), and an almost completely protein-non-permeable dialyzer, FX220 (Fresenius, Co. Ltd), in pre- and post-dilution HDF are compared in figure 3. The efficiency of high-molecular solutes removal by post-dilution HDF increased using either dialyzer, but long-term use was difficult due to increased albumin loss using BS-2.1UL. Therefore, BS-2.1UL is selected for pre-dilution HDF. On the other hand, AMG was not removed by pre-dilution HDF using FX220, showing that FX220 is inappropriate for pre-dilution HDF, but the albumin loss in post-dilution HDF was within the acceptable range, and, thus, the dialyzer is indicated for post-dilution HDF.

Selection of HPM Dialyzer for ol-HDF

Dialyzers used in previous large-scale studies on ol-HDF were only described as synthetic high-flux dialyzers, and only a few dialyzers were clearly presented. Dialyzers used in CONTRAST progressing in the multicenter study in Netherlands are clearly presented as FX80 (27%), FX100 (11%), OptifluxF200NR

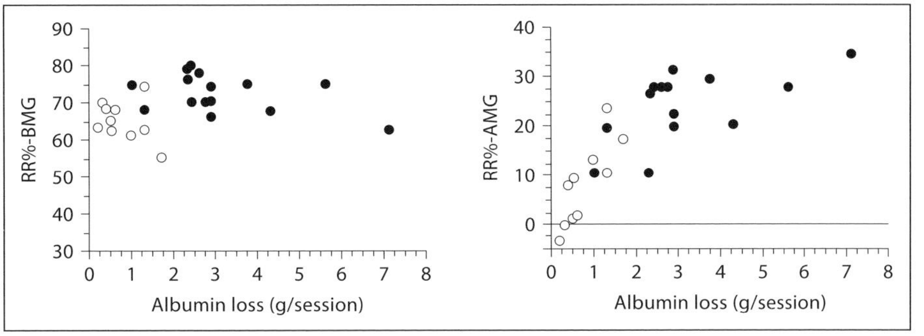

Fig. 4. Clinical data concerning the relationship between the BMG and AMG removal rates (RR%) and albumin loss in the HD mode of HPM dialyzers. Blood flow 200 ml/min, dialysate flow 500 ml/min, and dialysis time 240 min. ○ = IV type (BMG clearance >50 ml/min); ● = V type (BMG clearance >70 ml/min) HPM dialyzer. Data from proceedings of Japanese Society for HPM during 2006–2010.

(8%), Polyflux170H (25%), and Polyflux210H (27%) [13]. These correspond to type IV of the dialyzer performance classification in Japan (BMG clearance ≥50 ml/min, under conditions of blood flow 200 ml/min, and dialysate flow 500 ml/min). These possess sufficient BMG permeability, but are classified as non-protein-permeable dialyzers.

Regarding dialyzer performance necessary for ol-HDF, Canaud et al. [14] reported that a high-flux, high-performance dialyzer is required: the membrane should have a high hydraulic permeability (ultrafiltration coefficient: KUF >50 ml/h/mm Hg), high solute permeability (mass transfer-area coefficient: KoA urea >600 and BMG >60 ml/min), and large surface of exchange (1.5–2.1 m^2). These are mostly consistent with the requirements for type IV dialyzers in the Japanese classification.

The clinical data concerning the relationship between the BMG and AMG removal rates and albumin loss in the HD mode of HPM dialyzers put on the market over the last several years in Japan are shown in figure 4 (under the standard conditions in Japan, blood flow 200 ml/min, dialysate flow 500 ml/min, and dialysis time 240 min). The BMG removal rate and albumin loss were only weakly correlated, showing that a protein-permeable dialyzer is not necessary to remove substances with a molecular weight up to that of BMG. All these data were collected in the HD mode, showing that the current HPM dialyzers are sufficiently capable of removing substances in the BMG molecular weight range by HD mode.

In contrast, the AMG removal rate in the HD mode was well correlated with albumin loss, showing that the removal of substances in the AMG molecular weight range employing the HD mode results in excessive albumin loss.

The dilution method to be employed for each HPM dialyzer is clarified by applying these data to the HDF dilution method selection criteria described above. For example, a 2 g/session or greater albumin loss is capable of separating albumin loss and AMG removal when it is used for pre-dilution HDF.

HPM dialyzers are diverted for ol-HDF, as described above. However, performance in ol-HDF may markedly change due not only to the membrane performance, but also membrane diameter and dialyzer-housing shape. The development of devices exclusive for ol-HDF is necessary.

At the beginning of ol-HDF in Japan, the dialyzer performance corresponded to only type II-III type (BMG clearance < 50 ml/min) removal efficiency in the current dialyzer classification in Japan. Thus, elevation of the removal efficiency at a higher convective volume was attempted in ol-HDF, leading to its development. However, the performance of recent dialyzers has been markedly developed, and equivalent removal efficiency can now be achieved with non-ol-HDF. Accordingly, high-efficiency type IV or higher-grade dialyzers type V are now used for more than 90% of dialysis patients in Japan [15].

To demonstrate the efficacy of ol-HDF, it is necessary to compare conventional HD and ol-HDF using a type V dialyzer (BMG clearance ≥70 ml/min) widely employed in Japan, and re-investigate the significance of removing high-molecular solutes larger than BMG and protein-bound solutes.

Dialysis is performed using dialyzers with favorable biocompatibility and completely quality management dialysis fluid in Japan, reducing biological reactions on dialysis, and this condition is achievable by all dialysis facilities. Reconfirmation of the significance of ol-HDF in this dialysis environment may be necessary.

References

1 Goodkin DA, Bragg-Gresham JL, Koenig KG, Wolfe RA, Akiba T, Andreucci VE, Saito A, Rayner HC, Kurokawa K, Port FK, Held PJ, Young EW: Association of comorbid conditions and mortality in hemodialysis patients in Europe, Japan, and the United States: the Dialysis Outcomes and Practice Patterns Study (DOPPS). J Am Soc Nephrol 2003;14:3270–3277.

2 Sato T, Koga N: Centralized on-line hemodiafiltration system utilizing purified dialysate as substitution fluid. Artif Organs 1998;22: 285–290.

3 Kim ST: Characteristics of protein removal in hemodiafiltration. Contrib Nephrol. Basel, Karger, 1994, vol 108, pp 23–37.

4 Tsuchida K, Minakuchi J: Effect of large-size dialysis membrane and hemofiltration/hemodiafiltration methods on long-term dialysis patients. Contrib Nephrol. Basel, Karger, 2011, vol 168, pp 179–187.

5 Bammens B, Evenepoel P, Verbeke K, Vanrenterghem Y: Removal of the protein-bound solute P-cresol by convective transport: a randomized crossover study. Am J Kidney Dis 2004;44:278–285.

6 Masakane I: How to prescribe hemodialysis or hemodiafiltration in order to ameliorate dialysis-related symptoms and complications. Contrib Nephrol. Basel, Karger, 2011, vol 168, pp 53–63.

7 Ahrenholz P, Winkler RE, Ramlow W, Tiess M, Müller W: On-line hemodiafiltration with pre- and postdilution: a comparison of efficacy. Int J Artif Organs 1997;20:81–90.
8 Yamashita AC, Sakurai K: Choice of dialyzers for HDF. Contrib Nephrol. Basel, Karger, 2011, vol 168, pp 146–152.
9 Kim ST, Yamamoto C, Taoka M, Takasugi M: Programmed filtration, a new method for removing large molecules and regulating albumin leakage during hemodiafiltration treatment. Am J Kidney Dis 2001;38(suppl 1):S220–S223.
10 Vilar E, Fry AC, Wellsted D, Tattersall JE, Greenwood RN, Farrington K: Long-term outcomes in online hemodiafiltration and high-flux hemodialysis: a comparative analysis. Clin J Am Soc Nephrol 2009;4: 1944–1953.
11 Santoro A, Mancini E, Bolzani R, Boggi R, Cagnoli L, Francioso A, Fusaroli M, Piazza V, Rapanà R, Strippoli GF: The effect of online high-flux hemofiltration versus low-flux hemodialysis on mortality in chronic kidney failure: a small randomized controlled trial. Am J Kidney Dis 2008;52:507–518.
12 Locatelli F, Altieri P, Andrulli S, Bolasco P, Sau G, Pedrini LA, Basile C, David S, Feriani M, Montagna G, Di Iorio BR, Memoli B, Cravero R, Battaglia G, Zoccali C: Hemofiltration and hemodiafiltration reduce intradialytic hypotension in ESRD. J Am Soc Nephrol 2010;21:1798–807.
13 Penne EL, van der Weerd NC, Blankestijn PJ, van den Dorpel MA, Grooteman MP, Nubé MJ, Ter Wee PM, Lévesque R, Bots ML, CONTRAST Investigators: Role of residual kidney function and convective volume on change in β_2-microglobulin levels in hemodiafiltration patients. Clin J Am Soc Nephrol 2010;5:80–86.
14 Canaud B, Chenine L, Henriet D, Leray H: Online hemodiafiltration: a multipurpose therapy for improving quality of renal replacement therapy. Contrib Nephrol. Basel, Karger, 2008, vol 161, pp 191–198.
15 Nakai S, Suzuki K, Masakane I, Wada A, Itami N, Ogata S, Kimata N, Shigematsu T, Shinoda T, Syouji T, Taniguchi M, Tsuchida K, Nakamoto H, Nishi S, Nishi H, Hashimoto S, Hasegawa T, Hanafusa N, Hamano T, Fujii N, Marubayashi S, Morita O, Yamagata K, Wakai K, Watanabe Y, Iseki K, Tsubakihara Y: Overview of regular dialysis treatment in Japan (as of 31 December 2008). Ther Apher Dial 2010;14:505–540.

Hideki Kawanishi, MD
Tsuchiya General Hospital
3-30 Nakajima-cho, Naka-ku, Hiroshima 730-8655 (Japan)
Tel. +81 82 243 9191
E-Mail h-kawanishi@tsuchiya-hp.jp

Saito A, Kawanishi H, Yamashita AC, Mineshima M (eds): High-Performance Membrane Dialyzers.
Contrib Nephrol. Basel, Karger, 2011, vol 173, pp 44–52

Preferred Dialysis Fluid for the High-Performance Membrane

Tadashi Tomo

Department of Nephrology, Oita University Hospital, Oita University, Hasama-machi, Oita, Japan

Abstract

In the present study, we investigated the effect of hemodialysis (HD) with high-performance membrane filter (HPM-HD) using acetate-free bicarbonate dialysis (AFD) fluid on bioincompatibility as represented by inflammatory markers in patients undergoing maintenance HD therapy and compared it with conventional acetate-containing bicarbonate dialysis (ACD) fluid. A total of 36 maintenance HD patients were registered for study during the 4-month study period (22 males and 14 females, aged 63.5 ± 10.2 years, mean duration of dialysis 12.2 ± 8.6 years, chronic glomerular nephritis in 27 patients, diabetic nephropathy in 6 patients, and nephrosclerosis in 3 patients). These patients were subjected to ACD for the first 2 months followed by AFD fluid for the latter 2 months. Predialysis blood pH and bicarbonate were examined after each of the first and latter 2-month period. Blood variables of C-reactive protein (CRP) and interleukin-6 (IL-6) or fetuin-A were also determined. The filters (membrane surface area, raw material), the conditions of HD (blood flow rate, dialysate flow rate, dialysis time, dry weight) and drug regimen including erythrocyte-simulating agent (drug type, dosage) were unchanged throughout the study. There appeared to be significantly higher levels of predialysis blood pH and bicarbonate in the AFD phase than in the ACD phase. Blood CRP and IL-6 levels were significantly decreased in the AFD group as compared with those seen in the ACD group. From these results, it can be suggested that HPM-HD using AFD fluid contributes to correcting metabolic acidosis and alleviating microinflammation in HD patients.

Background

High-performance membrane filters (HPM) have a high permeability for substances ranging from small molecules to low-molecular-weight proteins. HPM also have a high biocompatibility. In dialysis therapy using these high permeable filters, backfiltration or backdiffusion is inevitable. Hence, the high biocompatibility of dialysis fluid is very important when using HPM. For several factors that influence the biocompatibility of dialysis fluid, the constituent of dialysis fluid is as important as the purity of dialysis fluid.

This study was undertaken to examine whether removal of acetate (contained at a concentration of 8–10 mEq/l in the conventional dialysis fluids) from the dialysis fluid or raising the concentration of HCO_3^- to 35 mEq/l (contained at a concentration of 30 mEq/l in the conventional dialysis fluids) would lead to alleviation of bioincompatible events as characterized by microinflammation observed during blood purification therapy or more efficient correction of metabolic acidosis in stable patients undergoing maintenance hemodialysis (HD). To this end, HPM-HD was carried out in these patients and thereby the effects of acetate-free bicarbonate dialysis (AFD) fluid were investigated and compared with conventional acetate-containing bicarbonate dialysis (ACD) fluid.

Purification of Dialysis Fluid

Purification of dialysis fluids is important when HPM are used because backfiltration or backdiffusion can occur. In Japan, the purity of dialysis fluids is defined by the following acceptable criteria [1]: (i) *bacterial counts:* not more than 0.1 CFU/ml, and (ii) *endotoxin (ET) level:* not more than 0.001 EU/ml (not more than the detectable limit).

Constituent of Dialysis Fluids

Buffer. Dialysis fluids currently used in Japan contain sodium bicarbonate as a buffer source. In the past, sodium acetate had been used as a buffer source because it was useful in avoiding precipitation of calcium carbonate from the dialysis fluid (likely to emerge if sodium bicarbonate is used) [2].

The adverse effects of acetate in HD patients have been known for the past several years and can be associated with intradialytic hypotension and cardiovascular instability; therefore, the primary buffer comprises bicarbonate in standard HD [3]. The bicarbonate-buffered dialysis fluids currently used in Japan contain small amounts of acetate as an additive to prevent crystallization of calcium and magnesium. Problems arising from such small amounts of acetate contained in the dialysis fluid have also been reported.

Electrolytes. The composition of dialysis fluids is fundamentally based on that of extracellular fluid, however individual electrolyte contained in dialysis fluids is somewhat unbalanced and is therefore required to be adjusted to a standard. Sodium concentration is set at 138–140 mEq/l, equivalent to that of extracellular fluid. Potassium in dialysis fluids is allowed to be set at a lower concentration of 2.0 mEq/l than that of extracellular fluid to correct hyperkalemia in HD patients with failure.

Glucose. A fasting blood glucose level is approximately 100 mg/dl in human blood, hence the use of a glucose-free dialysis fluid can incidentally cause

Table 1. Composition of dialysis fluids tested in the present study

	Na mEq/l	K mEq/l	Ca mEq/l	Mg mEq/l	Cl mEq/l	HCO_3^- mEq/l	Acetate mEq/l	Glucose g/l
Acetate (–) dialysate[1]	140	2.0	3.0	1.0	111	35	–	1.5
Acetate (+) dialysate	140	2.0	2.5	1.0	111	30	8	1.0

[1] Citrate 2 mEq/l is added.

hypoglycemia, aside from developing symptoms or not. Glucose in dialysis fluids is therefore contained so as to reach the final concentration of 100 mg/dl in the blood. It should be noted that hypoglycemia infrequently occurs even though such a glucose concentration is prepared because glucose is presumably metabolized in the body.

Methods

Patients

The study involved 36 HD patients in a stable clinical condition who were receiving HPM-HD (22 males and 14 females, aged 63.5 ± 10.2 years, mean duration of dialysis 12.2 ± 8.6 years). Primary diseases of renal failure were chronic glomerular nephritis in 27 patients, diabetic nephropathy in 6 patients, and nephrosclerosis in 3 patients. Informed consent was obtained from each patient prior to the study.

Conditions and Procedure for HD

HD was carried out 3 times weekly for 4–5 h/session at a blood flow rate of 200–250 ml/min and a dialysate flow rate of 500 ml/min. The compositions of ACD and AFD fluids tested in this study are presented in table 1. The purity and quality of the dialysis fluids was not more than 0.1 CFU/ml in terms of bacterial counts and not more than the detectable limit for the ET level at the end of the dialysis circuit.

The patients enrolled in this study, specified in the 'Patients' section, received treatment with ACD during the 2 months of the study followed by AFD during the latter 2 months. During the 4-month study period, comprising the first 2 months – the ACD phase (September 15 through November 15, 2009), and the latter 3 months – AFD phase (November 17 through January 15, 2010), only the dialysis fluid was changed, and the following conditions were kept unchanged: (1) filters (membrane surface area, raw material; table 2), (2) settings for HD, i.e. blood flow rate, dialysate flow rate, dialysis time, dry weight (3) drug regimen including erythrocyte-simulating agent (drug type, dosage). On the last Monday (for the Monday, Wednesday, and Friday dialysis group) or the last Tuesday (for the Tuesday, Thursday, and Saturday dialysis group) of each of the first and latter 2-month periods, blood was sampled from each patient.

Table 2. Type of dialysis membrane and conditions for HD

Case	Dialysis time, min	Blood flow rate, ml/min	Dialysis fluid rate, ml/min	Filter	Surface area, m^2	Raw material
1	300	250	500	PES-19Sα	1.9	polyethersulfone
2	300	250	500	APS-15SA	1.5	polysulfone
3	240	250	500	APS-21E	2.1	polysulfone
4	300	200	500	TS-1.6UL	1.6	polysulfone
5	300	250	500	VPS-15HA	1.5	polysulfone
6	300	250	500	VPS-15HA	1.5	polysulfone
7	270	200	500	FX-S220	2.2	polysulfone
8	300	250	500	APS-21E	2.1	polysulfone
9	330	250	500	APS-15SA	1.5	polysulfone
10	240	250	500	APS-15SA	1.5	polysulfone
11	270	250	500	FX-S220	2.2	polysulfone
12	270	250	500	APS-21E	2.1	polysulfone
13	300	250	500	APS-15E	1.5	polysulfone
14	270	250	500	APS-21E	2.1	polysulfone
15	300	250	500	FX-S220	2.2	polysulfone
16	240	250	500	PES-21Sα	2.1	polyethersulfone
17	300	200	500	H12-4000	1.53	polyacrylonitrile
18	300	250	500	APS-15SA	1.5	polysulfone
19	240	250	500	APS-21SA	2.1	polysulfone
20	270	250	500	APS-15SA	1.5	polysulfone
21	270	250	500	PES-21Sα	2.1	polyethersulfone
22	300	250	500	APS-18SA	1.8	polysulfone
23	180	250	500	TS-1.6UL	1.6	polysulfone
24	270	200	500	H12-4000	1.53	polyacrylonitrile
25	270	250	500	APS-15SA	1.5	polysulfone
26	270	200	500	APS-21E	2.1	polysulfone
27	300	250	500	PES-21Sα	1.2	polyethersulfone
28	270	200	500	ABH-18F	1.8	polysulfone
29	300	250	500	APS-18E	1.8	polysulfone

Table 2. Continued

Case	Dialysis time, min	Blood flow rate, ml/min	Dialysis fluid rate, ml/min	Filter	Surface area, m^2	Raw material
30	300	200	500	TS-1.6UL	1.6	polysulfone
31	300	250	500	TS-1.6UL	1.6	polysulfone
32	240	200	500	PES-21Sα	2.1	polyethersulfone
33	240	250	500	APS-18E	1.8	polysulfone
34	300	200	500	APS-18SA	1.8	polysulfone
35	300	250	500	ABH-18F	1.8	polysulfone
36	240	250	500	APS-15SA	1.5	polysulfone

Each blood sample was analyzed as follows: (1) C-reactive protein (CRP; SRL Co. Ltd), interleukin-6 (IL-6; R&D Systems, USA) and fetuin-A (Biovendor, Czech Republic) as markers related to inflammation. pH and HCO_3^- before the HD session were also analyzed.

Results

None of the 36 patients enrolled in this study developed any adverse event throughout the 4-month study period (first and later 2-month periods). This study was well tolerated for all patients with the following conditions to be kept unchanged: (1) settings for dialysis, i.e. the filter (membrane surface area, raw material), blood flow rate, dialysate flow rate, and dry weight; (2) drug regimen (drug type, dosage), and (3) erythrocyte-simulating agent (drug type, dosage).

Predialysis blood pH and bicarbonate levels were found to be significantly higher in the AFD phase than in the ACD phase ($p < 0.05$ and $p < 0.01$, respectively; table 3). AFD resulted in significant decreases in blood CRP levels as compared with the ACD fluid ($p < 0.05$; table 3). Such significantly lowered levels were also observed for IL-6 when the dialysis with AFD fluid was performed ($p < 0.05$; table 3). There was no significant difference in blood levels for fetuin-A in both the ACD fluid and AFD fluid ($p = 0.061$; table 3).

Discussion

Several adverse effects of acetate-buffered dialysis fluids due to acetate intolerance have been reported to be associated with higher cardiovascular risks leading to

Table 3. Comparison between conventional acetate-containing bicarbonate-buffered dialysis and acetate-free bicarbonate-buffered dialysis

	ACD (n = 36)	AFD (n = 36)	p
pH	7.369 ± 0.023	7.393 ± 0.036	<0.05
HCO_3^-, mEq/l	19.2 ± 2.3	21.1 ± 1.8	<0.01
IL-6, pg/ml	8.247 ± 7.08	5.594 ± 2.57	<0.05
CRP, mg/dl	0.21 ± 0.2	0.17 ± 0.17	<0.05
Fetuin-A, µg/ml	186.4 ± 43.8	196.9 ± 50.1	=0.061

Data are expressed as mean ± SD of 36 patients.
p values are shown as statistically significant level for comparison between ACD and AFD by paired t test.
ACD = Conventional acetate-containing bicarbonate-buffered dialysis; AFD = acetate-free bicarbonate-buffered dialysis.
Predialysis blood was sampled at the end of AFD and ACD phases during their respective 2-month periods.

the widespread use of bicarbonate-buffered dialysis fluids [2]. In Japan, some of the commercially available dialysis fluids are bicarbonate-buffered, which somewhat contain acetate (8–10 mEq/l) to prevent salt precipitation. So, this study was designed to explore the effects of HPM-HD therapy with AFD fluid on the prognostic factors for bioincompatible events including inflammation in HD patients, when compared with those with ACD fluid.

In predialysis analysis of blood pH and bicarbonate level, effective correction of metabolic acidosis was observed in the AFD phase evidenced by a significantly higher pH and bicarbonate level. It can be suggested that the effects depend on the relatively high concentrations of bicarbonate (35 mEq/l) contained in the AFD fluid. Lower predialysis blood levels of bicarbonate have been acknowledged to be associated with a higher risk of mortality for HD patients, and therefore it is recommended that the predialysis or stabilized serum should be maintained over 22 mEq/l by K/DOQI guidelines [4].

In the present study, the predialysis blood bicarbonate level was 21.1 ± 1.8 mEq/l in the AFD phase, which seems to fail to achieve K/DOQI guidelines. However, the values obtained in this study are the data collected on Monday or Tuesday, after an interdialytic interval of 2 days, whereas the criteria given in the K/DOQI guidelines pertain to the predialysis level obtained after an interdialytic interval of 1 day. Hence, one would conceive that, if blood sample in our study were taken after an interdialytic interval of 1 day, the values would satisfy the criteria specified in the K/DOQI guidelines. It is reported that correction of acidosis by administration of bicarbonate supplements reduces the phenylalanine efflux from leg tissues (muscle) in maintenance HD patients or improves nutritional status among patients with CKD [5, 6].

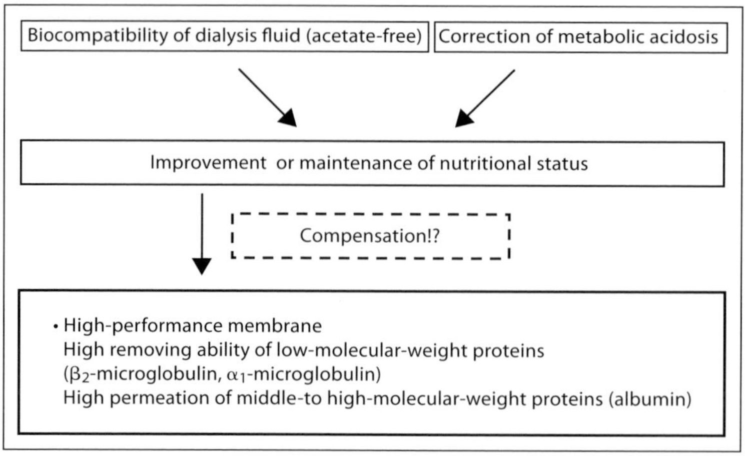

Fig. 1. Improvement or maintenance of nutritional status.

HPM has a high permeability for not only low-molecular-weight protein (as β_2-microglobulin, molecular weight (MW) 11,800) but also middle- to high-molecular-weight protein (as α_1-microglobulin, MW 33,000, or albumin, MW 66,000) [7]. In another report, online HDF using AFD improve the nutritional status in maintenance HD patients than in ACD phase [8]. Hence, in the case of HPM-HD, the efficient correction of metabolic acidosis leading to the improvement or maintenance of the nutritional status is very important (fig. 1).

Both CRP and IL-6, indicators of inflammatory reactions, seen during ACD, decreased significantly after being replaced by AFD. In the present study, the purity and quality of the dialysis fluids at the end of the dialysis circuit was consistently maintained below 0.1 CFU/ml in terms of bacterial count and below detectable limits for ET throughout the 4-month evaluation period. Furthermore, the conditional background for HPM-HD therapy including filter (membrane material, surface area), oral medication and erythrocyte-simulating agent (drug type, dosage) and settings for HD was kept unchanged, indicating that such situations are unlikely to affect CRP and IL-6 levels. Higuchi et al. [9] reported that cytokine production was significantly reduced during acetate-free biofiltration as compared with during dialysis with ACD, suggesting that the decreases in CRP and IL-6 observed in this study seem to reflect the influence of the absence of acetate in dialysis fluid. IL-6 can induce CRP [10], while the converse is also true, that is that in response to the reduction in IL-6, CRP production was downregulated in the present study. Both CRP and IL-6 have been reported to serve as predictors of the survival rates in maintenance HD patients, and lowered CRP and IL-6 levels can contribute to a better prognosis including survival advantage and improved clinical status [11].

Fetuin-A is a circulating calcium-regulatory glycoprotein that suppresses vascular and soft tissue calcification [12]. Fetuin-A reacts as a negative acute phase protein; downregulation is known to be associated with higher risk for mortality in HD patients [13, 14]. The present study showed that fetuin-A tended to be higher in the AFD phase than in the ACD phase, although not statistically significant.

The observation may be accounted for by alleviation of microinflammation found in the present study. In fact, Floege and Ketteler [15] reported that fetuin-A deficiency occurred in the presence of inflammation, and for the recovery, an intervention by administration of anti-inflammatory agents or steroid and purification of dialysis fluid was required. Based on the present study showing a decrease in CRP and IL-6, it can be assumed that elevated fetuin-A may be, at least partly, due to alleviation of inflammatory responses.

Limitations in the present study are the small number of subjects (36 patients) and inability to design a complete cross-over study (ACD→AFD→ACD). Sample size in our study had to be limited because it was relatively difficult to keep steady conditions such as dialysis settings and drug regimen for 4 months. The inability to execute a complete cross-over study is accounted for by the aspect that a central dialysis fluid delivery system (CDDS) is introduced in many Japanese medical facilities, namely if the dialysis fluid were changed for a cross-over study, patients other than the subjects of this study would be also involved. It should be considered that many of the 36 patients enrolled in our study strongly refused to resume ACD after AFD.

Conclusion

The results obtained in the present study indicate that the HPM-HD therapy with AFD fluid can significantly alleviate microinflammatory responses as compared with that with ACD fluid. Our data also suggest that even minimal amounts of acetate contained in the dialysis fluid can be bioincompatible for blood purification. HPM-HD with acetate-free dialysis fluid would be expected to improve the biocompatibility for dialysis therapy over conventional acetate-containing bicarbonate dialysis therapy. This improvement may do some good in contributing to the nutritional status in dialysis patients. Also, the efficient correction of metabolic acidosis is also important in improvement or maintenance of nutritional status in dialyzed patients.

In the case of HPM-HD accompanied with the permeation of protein, dialysis fluids with high biocompatibility or efficient ability for correction of metabolic acidosis are preferred.

References

1 Kawanishi H, Akiba T, Masakane I, Tomo T, Mineshima M, Kawasaki T, Hirakata H, Akizawa T: Standard on microbiological management of fluids for hemodialysis and related therapies by the Japanese Society for Dialysis Therapy 2008. Ther Apher Dial 2009;13:161–166.

2 Mion CM, Hegstrom RM, Boen ST, Scribner BH: Substitution of sodium acetate for sodium bicarbonate in the bath fluid for hemodialysis. Trans Am Soc Artif Intern Organs 1964;10:110–115.

3 Graefe U, Follette WC, Vizzo JE, Goodisman LD, Scribner BH: Reduction in dialysis-induced morbidity and vascular instability with the use of bicarbonate in dialysate. Proc Clin Dial Transplant Forum 1976;6:203–209.

4 National Kidney Foundation: K/DOQI clinical practice guidelines for nutrition in chronic renal failure. Am J Kidney Dis 2000; 35(suppl 2):S1–S140.

5 Löfberg E, Gutierrez A, Anderstam B, Wernerman J, Bergström J, Price SR, Mitch WE, Alvestrand A: Effect of bicarbonate on muscle protein in patients receiving hemodialysis. Am J Kidney Dis 2006;48:419–429.

6 De Brito-Ashurst I, Varagunam M, Raftery MJ, Yaqoob MM: Bicarbonate supplementation slows progression of CKD and improves nutritional status. J Am Soc Nephrol 2009;20: 2075–2084.

7 Tomo T, Matsuyama M, Nakata T, Kadota J, Toma S, Koga N, Fukui H, Arizono K, Takamiya T, Matsuyama K, Ueyama S, Shiohira Y, Uezu Y, Higa A: Effect of high fiber density ratio polysulfone dialyzer on protein removal. Blood Purif 2008;26: 347–353.

8 Matsuyama K, Tomo T, Kadota JI: Acetate-free blood purification can impact improved nutritional status in hemodialysis patients. J Artif Organs DOI 10.10007/s10047-010-0551-7.

9 Higuchi T, Yamamoto C, Kuno T, Okada K, Soma M, Fukuda N, Nagura Y, Takahashi S, Matsumoto K: A comparison of bicarbonate hemodialysis, hemodiafiltration, and acetate-free biofiltration on cytokine production. Ther Apher Dial 2004;8:460–467.

10 Weinhold B, Bader A, Poli V, Rüther U: Interleukin-6 is necessary, but not sufficient, for induction of the human C-reactive protein gene in vivo. Biochem J 1997;325: 617–621.

11 Stenvinkel P, Lindholm B: C-reactive protein in end-stage renal disease: are there reasons to measure it? Blood Purif 2005;23:72–78.

12 Ivanovski O, Drueke T, Massy ZA, Ketteler M, Floege J, Jahnen-Dechent W: Fetuin-A protects against atherosclerotic calcification in CKD. J Am Soc Nephrol 2009;20: 1264–1274.

13 Hermans MM, Brandenburg V, Ketteler M, et al: Netherlands Cooperative Study on the Adequacy of Dialysis (NECOSAD): association of serum fetuin-A levels with mortality in dialysis patients. Kidney Int 2007;72: 202–207.

14 Bláha V, Mistrík E, Dusilová-Sulková S: Circulating fetuin-A predicts early mortality in chronic hemodialysis patients. Clin Biochem 2009;42:996–1000.

15 Floege J, Ketteler M. Vascular calcification in patients with end-stage renal disease. Nephrol Dial Transplant 2004;19(suppl 5): V59–V66.

Tadashi Tomo, MD, PhD
Department of Nephrology
Oita University Hospital, Oita University
Hasama-machi, Oita 879-5593 (Japan)
Tel. +81 97 586 5804, E-Mail tomo@oita-u.ac.jp

Saito A, Kawanishi H, Yamashita AC, Mineshima M (eds): High-Performance Membrane Dialyzers.
Contrib Nephrol. Basel, Karger, 2011, vol 173, pp 53–57

Required Water Quality for the Use of High-Performance Membranes

Ikuo Aoike

Koyo Medical Clinic, Kameda-Koyo, Konan-Ku, Niigata, Japan

Abstract

The clinical benefits of high-performance membrane (HPM) dialyzers have often been reported since the advent of the synthetic polyacrylonitrile dialysis membrane. HPMs, which have high water permeability, eliminate a wide spectrum of uremic toxins, and offer excellent biocompatibility, are now essential for hemodialysis, hemofiltration, and hemodiafiltration. For HPMs whose mean pore size is enlarged to secure better dialysis membrane performance, however, the dialyzing fluid must be highly purified to prevent contamination. Blood purification therapies using highly purified dialyzing fluid and HPM are expected to improve the prognosis of future patients undergoing dialysis.

Improvement of Dialysis Membrane Performance

Cellulose dialysis membranes manufactured from cotton linters have long been used worldwide since the dawn of dialysis, because of the increased hydrophilic properties, excellent mechanical strength, and stable commercial supply. However, the classical and unmodified cellulose membranes exhibit poor permeability, and the majority of substances eliminated from the blood are of low molecular weight.

Under these conditions, the risk of backdiffusion of pyrogens and other dialysis fluid contaminants into the blood compartment was presumably minimal. As if in response to the middle-molecule hypothesis proposed by Babb et al. [1], polyacrylonitrile (PAN) membranes, a plate-type synthetic polymer membrane with higher permeability, appeared in 1973, leading to the widespread use of larger pore dialysis membranes. Profound cases of transient leukopenia were observed during dialysis with cellulosic membranes [2]. These were the result of complement activation by cellulosic membranes [3]. However, PAN membranes caused less severe cases of transient leukopenia than cellulosic membranes, and the excellent biocompatible characteristics of the synthetic polymer membranes were thereby demonstrated. The cause of the dialysis-related amyloidosis was identified in 1985 as 11,800-Da β_2-microglobulin [4]. Since then, β_2-microglobulin and other low-molecular-weight proteins have become the target uremic toxins for dialytic removal. Synthetic hollow-fiber membranes, such as PAN, polysulfone, and polymethylmethacrylate, were extensively modified to improve the elimination characteristics for low-molecular-weight proteins, as well as water permeability. The most effective way was to increase the pore size of the membrane. Consequently, such endeavors led to the widespread use of synthetic polymer dialysis membranes that are excellent in removal, water permeability, and biocompatibility. High-performance membrane (HPM)-based hemodialysis treatment has significantly improved prognosis [5], curbed the incidence of dialysis-related amyloidosis [6–8], and yielded other clinical benefits.

Compatibility with Various Dialysis Modalities

HPMs are used not only for routine hemodialysis but for hemodiafiltration requiring substitution fluid because of high permeability, push-pull hemodiafiltration, online hemodiafiltration infusing large volumes of substitution fluid, and simple hemofiltration. Because the hydrostatic dialysis fluid pressure exceeds the hydrostatic blood pressure at the blood outlet port of the hemodiafiltration system, backfiltration from the dialysis fluid into the blood compartment occurs. The internal filtration-enhanced hemodialysis system provides effects similar to hemodiafiltration by elevating the backfiltration rate within the dialyzer [9].

Importance of the Dialysis Fluid Quality

Baz et al. [10] reported in 1991 that the use of ultrapure dialysis fluid with low endotoxin levels reduced the incidence of dialysis-related amyloidosis. They found that the incidence of dialysis-related amyloidosis was decreased in patients undergoing dialysis with cellulose-based membranes and ultrapure dialysis fluid. For dialysis with HPMs, which have a mean pore size larger than that of cellulosic membranes, the biological and chemical purity of the dialysis fluid has been shown to impact the quality of the dialysis treatment. Schwalbe et al. [11] found that a more frequent use of reverse osmosis water resulted in a lower prevalence of dialysis-related amyloidosis. The Schwalbe study underscores the importance of the purity of dialysis fluid.

Dialysis Fluid Contamination Markers

Biological contamination of dialysis fluid primarily relates to viruses, Gram-positive and -negative bacteria, fungi, and other exogenous pyrogens. Testing methods commonly applied for detecting dialysis fluid contaminants of biological origin include culture tests for aquatic microbes and the measurements of endotoxin components of the Gram-negative bacterial cell wall. In culture tests for aquatic microbes, samples are placed on R2A or TGEA media, and incubated at 17–23°C for 7 days.

Bacterial endotoxins generally have a molecular weight of several hundred thousand daltons, and form micelles in water because they have both hydrophilic and hydrophobic regions. Such large-molecular-weight solutes do not pass through intact dialysis membranes, however the endotoxin fragments of several thousands to several ten thousand daltons that permeate from the dialysis fluid into the blood circulation raise clinical concern. The endotoxin contamination criteria have been determined for the *Limulus* test. Other markers of dialysis fluid contaminants include microparticles, TOC (total organic carbon), silica, etc.

Mechanism of Blood Contamination by Dialysis Fluid

The major route of removal of various substances is diffusion across the dialysis membrane between the blood and dialysis fluid compartments. Classical cellulose-based membranes are unlikely to achieve a sufficient blood-to-dialysis fluid diffusion gradient even for substances of low molecular weight. In addition, they are unlikely to facilitate backdiffusion of these substances. However, HPMs having a large pore size allow untoward rapid diffusion of dialyzed endotoxin fragments back into the blood compartment. Analysis of the intradialyzer pressure distribution indicates that the dialysis fluid flows back into blood circulation in the region of the blood outlet port, thereby presenting the risk of direct blood contamination. Endotoxin fragments are known to be adsorbed onto polysulfone and polyamide filters. In particular, polymethylmethacrylate, which has an excellent adsorption profile for low-molecular-weight proteins, has been demonstrated to capture endotoxins quite effectively [12]. Based on these considerations, the purification of the dialysis fluid is a critical condition for effective HPM dialysis.

Dialysis Water Criteria

The American Association for Medical Instrumentation (AAMI) and the *European Pharmacopoeia* established in the 1990s the biological and chemical contamination criteria for hemodialysis water treatment. Since 2004, the discussions have been held for establishing new International Organization for Standardization (ISO) guidelines, based on the American National Standards Institute (ANSI)-AAMI RD52 standard. In Japan, the Japanese Society for Dialysis Therapy launched the dialysis safety standards in 1996, the safety guidelines for dialysis fluid prepared by and medical institutions installing the AK100 Ultra system in 1998, and the standard on microbiological management of fluids in Japanese Society for Dialysis Therapy in 2008 [13]. In order to meet these water safety requirements in Japan, it is important to develop and implement the dialysis fluid management system, including the use of endotoxin-retentive filters, for facilities running the central dialysis fluid delivery system (constituting the majority of Japanese dialysis facilities), as well as those employing single-patient dialysis machines [14].

Future Expectation for HPM Dialysis with Highly Purified Dialysis Fluid

The use of highly purified dialysis fluid has been reported to yield various clinical advantages: a reduction in the dose of erythropoiesis-stimulating agents for the treatment of renal anemia, suppression of dialysis-related amyloidosis, improvement in pruritus, reduced levels of interleukin-6 and C-reactive proteins, and alleviation of oxidative stress symptoms. In addition, the positive relationship between improvements in malnutrition-inflammation-atherosclerosis syndrome and the purity of the dialysis fluid has been pointed out [15]. These significant clinical effects are unlikely the result of purification alone. Other factors, such as the excellent biocompatibility of the dialyzer membrane materials, high water permeability of the dialyzer, and the removal of a wide spectrum of uremic toxins, seem to contribute in a synergistic manner.

Conclusion

HPMs play an important role in the various dialysis treatment modalities available today, due to the high water permeability, capability to remove a wide range of uremic toxins, excellent biocompatibility, and other characteristic features. However, because of the large pore size, HPMs are likely to allow blood to be contaminated by the dialysis fluid. HPM hemopurification therapies using highly purified dialysis fluid will significantly improve the prognosis of dialysis patients.

References

1 Babb AL, Farrell PC, Uvelli DA, Scribner BH: Hemodialyzer evaluation by examination of solute molecular spectra. Trans Am Soc Artif Intern Organs 1972;18:98–105, 122

2 Koplow LS, Goffinet JA: Profound neutropenia during the early phases of hemodialysis. JAMA 1968,203:1135–1137.

3 Craddock PR, Fehr J, Dalmasso AP, et al: Hemodialysis leukopenia: pulmonary vascular leukostasis resulting from complement activation by dialyzer cellophane membrane. J Clin Invest 1977, 59:879–888.

4 Gejyo F, Yamada T, Odani S, Nakagawa Y, Arakawa M, Kunitomo T, Kataoka H, Suzuki M, Hirasawa Y, Shirahama T: A new form of amyloid protein associated with chronic hemodialysis was identified as β_2-microglobulin. Biochem Biophys Res Commun 1985;129:3 701–706.

5 Koda Y, Nishi S, Miyazaki S, et al: Switch from conventional to high flux membrane reduces the risk of carpal tunnel syndromes and mortality of hemodialysis patients. Kidney Int 1997;52:1096–1101.

6 Chanard J, Bindi P, Lavaud S, et al: Carpal tunnel syndrome and type of dialysis membrane. BMJ 1989;298:867–868.

7 Van Ypersele de Strihou C, Jadoul M, Malghem J, et al: The working party on dialysis amyloidosis. Kidney Int 1991;39: 1012–1019,

8 Aoike I, Gejyo F, Arakawa M, Kataoka H, Kunitomo T, Hakim RM: Niigata Research Programme for β_2M Removal Membrane: Ten-year follow-up multicentre clinical trial of PMMA membrane dialysis. ERA-EDTA Abstr 299, 1999.

9 Dellanna F, Wuepper A, Baldamus CA: Internal filtration – advantage in haemodialysis? Nephrol Dial Transplant 1996;11(suppl 2):83–86.

10 Baz M, Durand C, Jaber K, Andrieu D, et al: Using ultrapure water in hemodialysis delays carpal tunnel syndrome. Int Artif Organs 1991;14:681–685.

11 Schwalbe S, Holzhauer M, Schaeffer J, et al: Beta-2-microglobulin-associated amyloidosis: a vanishing complication of long-term hemodialysis? Kidney Int 1997;52: 1077–1083.

12 Cappelli G, Ballestri M, Di Felice A, Bonucchi D, Albertazza A: Pyrogen transfer across PMMA membrane. Contrib Nephrol. Basel, Karger, 1998, vol 125, pp 233–239.

13 Kawanishi H, Akiba T, Masakane I, Tomo T, Mineshima M, Kawasaki T, Hirakata H, Akizawa T: Standard on microbiological management of fluids for hemodialysis and related therapies by the Japanese Society for Dialysis Therapy 2008. Ther Apher Dial 2009;3:161–166.

14 Aoike I: Characteristics of central dialysis fluid delivery system and single patient dialysis machine for HDF. Contrib Nephrol. Basel, Karger, 2011, vol 168, pp 99–106.

15 Stenvinkle P, Heimburger O, Lindholm B, et al: Are there two types of malnutrition in chronic renal failure? Evidence for relationships between malnutrition, inflammation, and atherosclerosis (MIA syndrome). Nephrol Dial Transplant 2000;15:953–960.

Ikuo Aoike
Koyo Medical Clinic
3-9-25 Kameda-Koyo, Konan-ku
Niigata 950-0121 (Japan)
Tel. +81 25 385 8686, E-Mail kmc8686@an.wakwak.com

Saito A, Kawanishi H, Yamashita AC, Mineshima M (eds): High-Performance Membrane Dialyzers.
Contrib Nephrol. Basel, Karger, 2011, vol 173, pp 58–69

Clinical Outcomes of the High-Performance Membrane Dialyzer

Yutaka Koda

Koda Medical and Dialysis Clinic, Tsubame, Niigata, Japan

Abstract

HPM (high-performance membrane or high-flux membrane) has better biocompatibility and higher capacity to remove retention solutes of large molecular weight, which has been proven to be toxic especially to cardiovascular and skeletal organs. To date, several non-randomized observational studies have shown a reduction in morbidity and mortality in HPM-treated patients compared with low-flux conventional membrane. Meanwhile, two randomized controlled trials were unable to reveal the superiority of high-flux membrane in survival of all-cause mortality, but suggested a significant benefit by subgroup analyses or post-hoc analyses in patients with diabetes, hypoalbuminemia and long duration of prior dialysis. Thus, the results of the published studies are conflicting and it still cannot be explained whether the effect is based on the biocompatibility of the membrane or on the differences in the clearance of middle molecules, or on the microbiological purity of dialysate which improved simultaneously with the flux increment. As survival outcome might be determined by additional multiple confounding factors, dialysis-related or non-dialysis-related, investigations to control them are difficult to perform. Although the clinical results are non-conclusive and it is still unanswered how much large molecule removal is required to improve outcomes in routine clinical practice, there is a considerable amount of biological plausibility for high-flux dialysis or middle molecule removal. Further trials will be required to confirm what patient group benefits the most, the magnitude of advantages and how large the molecules are and how much molecule removal is acceptable using advanced high-performance dialyzers. Dispersing hazardous effects by a low-quality therapy should be taken more seriously than practicing a high-quality therapy of uncertain superiority.

Conceptual Meaning of High-Performance Membrane Dialyzer

The description of membrane as high-flux or low-flux is primarily based on hydraulic permeability, but currently is based on the ability to remove large solutes like β_2-microglobulin (B2M). A high-performance membrane (HPM) dialyzer is one containing a high-flux membrane conceptually aspired to native kidney performance, and is currently regarded as allowing excellent removal of large molecules (B2M or larger than B2M including albumin to an acceptable level) with better biocompatibility closer to the natural kidney filter. At present, such a membrane is mostly synthetic (PS, PMMA, PAN, PEPA, PES, PAES, PA), except cellulose triacetate. Device design is another crucial factor for determining performance such as inner diameter, effective length, waving, and filling ratio of the hollow fiber to modify blood and dialysate path resistance.

Background of Developing HPM Dialyzers in Japan

The policy to treat end-stage renal disease patients with CKD-5 who need blood purification therapy varies considerably from one country to the other. In Japan, kidney transplantation has been performed in a quite restricted number of patients, probably because of a religious dilemma or scientists' inattentive attitude towards the brain death dispute. It followed that the number of hemodialysis patients with very long-term dialysis has increased at an accelerated rate every year, reaching up to nearly 290,675; at the end of 2009, 3.7% of them had been on dialysis for over 25 years. Among the patients alive in 2009, the longest dialysis duration recorded is 41.8 years [1].

Cardiovascular problems, malnutrition, and dialysis-related amyloidosis (DRA) are common in such long-term dialysis patients, attending for physical disability and morbidity. With a decrease in residual renal function, retention of middle molecules may occur. Uremic toxicity of these large molecules has been revealed to play a role, especially in the pathogenesis of these long-term dialysis morbidities [2]. Unfortunately, no remedy for DRA has been found, although a successful kidney transplant may stop the disease from progressing. It has increasingly become a serious problem because it not only affects the musculoskeletal system but also internal organs. Therefore, DRA has caught the attention of dialysis engineers who are striving to develop new dialysis membranes that can remove large amounts of B2M from the blood.

Based on the above background, the HPM dialyzer, a high-flux dialyzer with better performance, has been the major research project to ameliorate these comorbid illnesses and to improve the outcome of the patients.

An annual HPM conference has been held for over 35 years since the discovery of DRA. The conference offers a platform to exchange information, repeating the consecutive process of announcing new HPM dialyzers by the manufacturers, reporting the clinical experience of users and then introducing an improved version a year later. It has created a virtuous feedback loop for rapid development of membranes with a higher performance level.

Middle molecule removal has been improved by the introduction of large-pore membranes added along with enhanced filtration within the dialyzer (internal filtration). Recent HPM dialyzers utilize the internal filtration and permeate larger molecules up to near albumin size, aiming at removal of larger and protein-bound uremic toxins. Combining these mechanisms, some HPM dialyzers exert B2M clearance up to nearly 80 ml/min, which is comparable with convective therapy like hemofiltration or hemodiafiltration [3]. High-flux dialysis with enhanced internal filtration does not need a complex machine and thus is more cost-effective in view of large solute removal [4].

There are caveats though in using such high-performance membranes. Excessive pressure load and ultrafiltration in the arterial part of the dialyzer induces unpredictable albumin leakage and fouling of the membrane's surface. The dissociations between hydraulic permeability and solute permeability pose the problem that the removal characteristics differ extremely depending on how they are used [5]. It demonstrates the necessity for independent measures for large solute removal properties for each dialyzer by various modes of use.

Survival Outcomes and Membrane Choice

Clinical influences of large pore membrane have been previously reported to give a beneficial effect on DRA, dyslipidemia, inflammation, malnutrition, residual renal function, infection and insulin resistance [6]. These effects and pathophysiology linking dialyzer membrane are still controversial and could not be completely ascertained. However, it is tempting to speculate that these clinical benefits could contribute to improve the mortality which remains unacceptably high in hemodialysis patients compared with the general population.

In the 1990s, several retrospective observational studies showed a reduction in morbidity and mortality in patients on high-flux dialysis compared with low-flux dialysis (table 1). In reports by Hornberger et al. [7] and Koda et al. [8], a sophisticated method was adopted using a time-dependent covariate in the Cox proportional hazard model, though the method had a problem in adjusting the carry-over effect of prior therapy. Hakim et al. [9] reported a 20% reduction of mortality by using biocompatible membrane compared with unmodified cellulose membrane. Bloembergen et al. [10] also reported less infection and less coronary artery disease based on the same membrane classification as Hakim's report [9]. Leypoldt et al. [11] reported that a 10% increase in vitamin B_{12} (1,355 Da) clearance by the dialyzer was associated with a 5% decrease in mortality in a retrospective analysis, even when urea Kt/V was held constant. It suggests that differences in mortality when using different types of membrane may be explained by differences in middle molecule removal.

Contrary to these results, some authors reported no influence of membrane on mortality. Bonomini et al. [12] found no difference in survival between the

Table 1. Reports on RR of mortality compared with high-dialysis with low-flux dialysis [7–20, 26]

Author	Comparison	Study design	Report	RR	n	p value
Hornberger	C vs. PS	O, Retro	1992	0.24	253	<0.001
Chandran	regenerated C vs. PAN (AN-69)	O, Retro	1993	deaths: 203 vs. 132	352	<0.001
Bonomini	C vs. synth.	O, Retro	1995	no difference	122	NS
Locatelli	Lf (C,PS) vs. Hf PS (HD, HDF)	RCT	1996	no difference	205	NS
Hakim	unmod. C vs. mod. C/synth	O, Retro	1996	0.80	2,410	<0.045
Koda	Hf (HD, HDF) vs. Lf	O, Retro	1997	0.61	819	<0.05
Leypoldt	membranes grouped by vitamin B_{12} clearance	O, Retro	1999	0.953[1]	1,771	<0.0001
Bloembergen	unmod. C vs. mod. C/synth	O, Retro	1999	0.82	4,055	<0.002
Woods	Hf PS vs. Lf PS	O, Retro	2000	0.58	715	<0.029
Port	Hf synth vs. Lf synth	O, Retro	2001	0.81	4,448	<0.04
HEMO, Eknoyan	Hf vs. Lf	RCT	2002	0.92	1,846	NS
HEMO, Cheung (HD >3.7 years)	Hf vs. Lf	RCT, subgroup analysis	2003	0.68	577	<0.005
Chauveau	Hf vs. Lf	O, Pro	2005	0.62	650	0.03
Canaud	Hf vs. Lf	O, Pro	2006	1.03	1,912	NS
Krane (type 2 diabetes)	Hf synth vs. Lf C	O, Retro	2007	0.24	285	<0.0001
	Hf synth vs. Lf semisynth	O, Retro	2007	0.45	360	<0.0001
	Hf synth vs. Lf synth	O, Retro	2007	0.63	488	<0.0006
Yokoyama	Hf vs. Lf	O, Pro	2008	0.72	1,207	NS
MPO, Locatelli	Hf vs. Lf	RCT	2009	0.76	647	NS, 0.09

Table 1. Continued

Author	Comparison	Study design	Report	RR	n	p value
MPO, Locatelli (albumin <4.0 g/dl, DM)	Hf vs. Lf	RCT, subgroup analysis	2009	0.63	493	0.01

RR is transformed as low flux assumed to be 1.0 in this table.
Historical prospective study is classified into retrospective cohort.
n = Sample number; O = observational study; Retro = retrospective cohort study; Pro = prospective cohort study. NS = statistically not significant; C = cellulose; Hf = high-flux; Lf = low-flux; RC = regenerated cellulose; mod. C = modified cellulose; unmod. C = unmodified cellulose; PS = polysulfone; PAN = polyacrylonitrile = PMMA = polymethylmethacrylate; synth = synthetic membrane; RCT = randomized controlled study; HEMO study = Hemodialysis Membrane Outcome Study; MPO = Membrane Permeability Outcome Study.
[1] By 10% increase of vitamin B_{12} clearance.

groups in a small-sized retrospective study without adjustment for comorbidity. Locatelli et al. [13] in a 2-year prospective study with random assignment to low-flux dialysis (biocompatible and bioincompatible), high-flux dialysis and hemodiafiltration did not find significant differences in morbidity and mortality among them; however, the primary aim of the study was not to detect mortality.

To address the unanswered question about the outcome benefit of high-flux membranes, two randomized controlled trials (RCTs) were conducted in the 2000s, the Hemodialysis (HEMO) study in prevalent patients and the Membrane Permeability Outcome (MPO) study in incident patients. The HEMO study was the largest RCT (n = 1,846) ever to determine whether increasing the dose of dialysis or using a high-flux dialyzer alters survival or morbidity among hemodialysis patients. A primary analysis of the HEMO study did not show a major benefit of all-cause mortality, but a reduction of risk for cardiac-related events was observed in patients randomly assigned to high-flux membranes [14]. In a secondary analysis, the influence of prior dialysis duration on clinical outcomes of high-flux dialysis was investigated. A significantly lower risk was observed in the high-flux arm of the long dialysis duration group (8.6 ± 4.9 years) in all-cause mortality (relative risk [RR] 0.68) and cardiac death (RR 0.63) [15]. Cheung et al. [16] suggested that mortality was inversely related to predialysis B2M levels in subanalysis of the HEMO study. We confirmed that the use of HPM with filtered dialysate (ET <0.06 EU/ml in 1995) obviously reduced predialysis B2M in both incident and prevalent patients (fig. 1a, b) and was presumed advantageous in survival outcome [8]. B2M levels are the result of

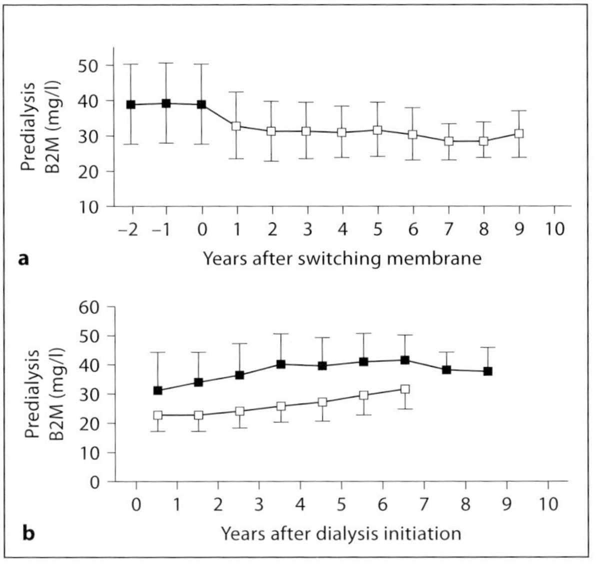

Fig. 1. Time course of predialysis B2M concentrations in patients with high-flux (□) and low-flux membrane (■). Lower levels are maintained in both (**a**) prevalent patients (n = 181) and (**b**) incident patients (n = 357) by high-flux dialysis [8].

both clearance and sustained inflammation. We speculate that both an enhancement of large molecule removal and ETRF-filtered dialysate suppressed B2M generation, thus contributing to maintain lower predialysis B2M levels. These reports indicate the association of middle molecules in mortality but not the cause-effect relationship.

A MPO study conducted in several European centers from 1998 to 2003 [17] enrolled only incident patients, avoiding a carry-over effect of prior therapy with low-flux dialyzers and minimizing survival bias (selection of survivors). The overall analysis did not show a survival advantage for high-flux membrane as the HEMO study did, but subgroup analysis showed significantly higher survival rates in the high-flux subgroup of patients with a serum albumin <4 g/dl (RR 0.63) and the diabetic group ($p = 0.039$, Kaplan-Meier analysis).

These two large RCTs failed to reveal a survival benefit of high-flux dialysis in primary analysis, but in a post-hoc analysis it may benefit at least some groups of patients. Further observational studies in the mid-2000s agreed with the results of these subgroup analyses of RCT. Chauveau et al. [18] found a significant survival benefit of high-flux membranes in long-term patients whose time on dialysis (8.5 ± 6.0 years) was closely similar to the HEMO study in a 30-month prospective follow-up of a non-randomized cohort. It is suggested that all-cause mortality depends on the duration of prior dialysis corresponding to the HEMO study. The 4D study evaluated atorvastatin in high-risk patients (diabetes and hemodialysis) and considered post hoc the patients who were treated with the same membrane type during the entire follow-up period [19]. The RR of mortality in diabetes patients treated with synthetic low-flux membrane was 59% greater than in those who were treated with synthetic high-flux membranes. Thus the same observational study results are consistent with RCT secondary analyses, particularly in subgroups of patients with long-term dialysis or diabetes. Taken together, the above-mentioned results suggest that membrane flux rather than biocompatibility may influence mortality in dialysis patients.

In contrast, a Japanese prospective cohort study published in 2008 showed no benefit of biocompatibility or permeability of membranes to anemia and mortality [20]. But in this study, the definition of a high-flux dialyzer with a B2M clearance of GT 10 ml/min seems too low at present. Most high-flux dialyzers in Japan currently demonstrate a B2M clearance of >60 ml/min and even in the HEMO study it was on average 33.8 ml/min [14]. The actual predialysis B2M levels of each group are not stated in the report, indicating an uncertain effect of high-flux dialysis. A relatively low dialyzer performance may explain the negative result.

There is another noteworthy observation of biocompatibility and permeability. Charra et al. [21] have reported the best long-term survival data in the world. This outstanding survival might be attributed to long hours of dialysis and a high Kt/V with excellent blood pressure control. It is interesting to note that a complement-activating membrane and acetate dialysate were exclusively used in their cohort. This suggests membrane is less important than the dose of dialysis or blood pressure control. But by rough comparison of Kaplan-Meier analysis between Charra's and Koda's cohort, the survival after 15 years seems to be superior in the latter that switched to the treatment with high-flux biocompatible membrane and ultrafiltered bicarbonate dialysate [22]. This suggests that high-flux dialysis with purified dialysate has a role in preventing life-threatening complications specifically occurring after long-term dialysis.

Ward [23] indicates in his review the importance of dialysis prescription rather than choice of membrane, such as length and frequency of treatments, for outcome improvement. Because flux performance has currently reached limits of multicompartmental behavior or the protein-bound nature of toxins, it hampers efficient removal even by maximally upgraded clearance. A comprehensive and combined approach must always be essential for better outcome.

Close Association between Biocompatibility, Flux and Dialysate Purity

Membrane classification by biocompatibility is ambiguous for the close association of biocompatibility and solute removal. Classification of dialyzers as being biocompatible or bioincompatible is usually based on complement activation or leukopenia. But this classification is too simplistic because of the many other criteria that can be used to judge biocompatibility, like thrombogenicity, sterilization, and so on. Recently, oxidative stress by immune cell stimulation has been emphasized to play a role in long-term consequences which produce advanced glycation end-products, advanced lipoxidation end-products and advanced oxidation protein products. At present no dialysis membrane can be absolutely inert. Additionally the flux itself modifies biocompatibility by removing anaphylatoxins by diffusion or adsorption to the membrane, posing a caveat when interpreting the relationship between biocompatibility and clinical outcome [24]. In addition, dialysate purity considerably affects the chronic inflammatory state of the dialysis patient. Thus it would be extremely complex and difficult to compare outcomes by biocompatibility classification.

Although there is no distinct evidence, dialysate purity should particularly be emphasized in patients using HPM, because backfiltration of dialysate cannot be avoided in high-flux dialysis. The use of ultrapure dialysate was associated with lower proinflammatory cytokines and acute phase proteins, thus contributing to relieving the long-term morbidity of maintenance dialysis patients. The main impacts are improvement of nutritional status, erythropoietin responsiveness, uremic dyslipidemia, delaying the onset of DRA and preservation of residual renal function [25].

Despite the use of high-flux dialyzers, only a few reports on survival have referred to dialysate purity in particular. Patients were treated with ultrafiltered dialysate with endotoxin levels <20 pg (0.06 EU)/ml in Koda's report [8] and <0.25 EU/ml in Woods' report [26], which might have prevented inflammation triggering by backfiltration of high-flux dialysis. Dialysate purity is the premise to use HPM dialyzers. When interpreting an outcome study of high-flux dialysis, it must be confirmed whether the dialysate was purified or not. It is now recommended in Europe and Japan to use ultrapure dialysate for all patients with high-flux dialysis.

Interpretation of Proof of Quality and Demand for Further RCTs

A prospective RCT is the only method to provide a golden standard, but a RCT would not always be possible to conduct from an ethical point of view. In a series of experimental studies, evidence about biocompatibility and flux has already suggested the biological plausibility of a high-flux biocompatible membrane. The scientific, unbiased analysis (i.e. to examine the hypothesis) and the problems connected directly with patients' interest (i.e. to find the better therapy) could be distinguished. The difference of the evidence level might be accepted between an explanatory study and pragmatic study in a clinical setting.

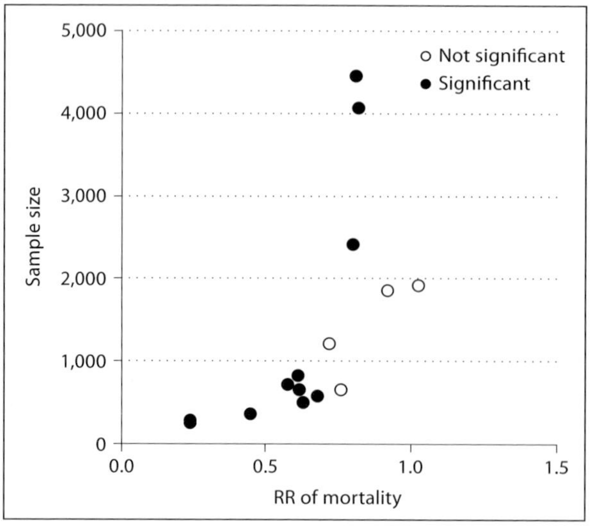

Fig. 2. A scatter plot of treatment effect (RR of mortality) against a measure of study size (funnel plot). The funnel is visually near symmetric, but suggests publication bias is still likely on the side of negative results. A higher effect in a small study size might also suggest selection bias or intensive intervention. RR of mortality is adopted from the lists shown in table 1. Low-flux membrane is assumed to be 1.

As mortality is a total result of complicated factors and there are so many confounders to be adjusted, RR reduction will be considerably variable among studies. A funnel plot is a scatter plot of treatment effect against a measure of study size. It is used primarily as a visual aid for detecting bias or systematic heterogeneity. An asymmetric funnel indicates the possibility of either publication bias or a systematic difference between smaller and larger studies (small study effects).

A funnel diagram based on the papers listed in table 1 suggests publication bias is still likely on the side of negative results (fig. 2). A higher effect in a small study size might also suggest selection bias or intensive intervention. More RCTs of a large sample size are needed in order to determine the truth of RR of mortality.

There is a difference in degree of interest and enthusiasm among countries to remove middle molecules. It may come from differences of the patient's background such as years on dialysis, prevalence of kidney transplantation and the financial issues of the health insurance system. European Best Practice Guidelines for Hemodialysis recommend high-flux membranes with specific indications [27]. Japanese hemodialysis patients are now on high-flux membranes in an overwhelming 97% of cases [28] and 11.4% are on protein-permeable membrane with B2M clearance >70 ml/min. In contrast, NKF/DOQI comments are rather indefinite and unmodified cellulose dialyzer membranes for dialysis are discouraged [29].

Conclusion

To date, no unequivocal evidence is available supporting that biocompatible high-flux membranes are definitely superior to low-flux membranes. However, the results of some studies support the use of high-flux membranes in some populations to improve survival, especially in such patients with diabetes, long prior dialysis and hypoalbuminemia. To clarify HPM contributions to patient outcome, it may be necessary to enroll more long-term dialysis patients (>15 years), to apply a more strengthened dialyzer (B2M clearance >70 ml/min or more) and to use ultrapure dialysate as a routine practice, that is, clarification of the therapeutic object and the treatment intensity. Natural kidney obviously eliminates not only small solutes like urea but also large molecules up to low-molecular-weight proteins. Until now, no report has been found that insists low-flux dialysis provides better survival than high-flux dialysis. Dispersing hazardous effects by a low-quality therapy should be taken more seriously than practicing a high-quality therapy of uncertain superiority.

References

1 Registry of Japanese Society for Dialysis Therapy (RJSDT): An overview of regular dialysis treatment in Japan as of December 31, 2009. Tokyo, RJSDT, 2009.

2 Vanholder RC: Advantages of new hemodialysis membranes and equipment. Nephron Clin Pract 2010;114:c165–c172.

3 Kudo T: Polysulfone membrane; in Takesawa S, et al (eds): High-Performance Membrane Dialyzers, 2008 (in Japanese). Tokyo, Igakusha, 2008, pp 37–48.

4 Koda Y: Internal filtration-enhanced hemodialysis is a cost-effective treatment in view of solute removal. Blood Purif 2004;22 (suppl 2):36–39.

5 Ahrenholz PG, Winkler RE, Michelsen A, Lang DA, Bowry SK: Dialysis membrane-dependent removal of middle molecules during hemodiafiltration: the β_2-microglobulin/albumin relationship. Clin Nephrol 2004;62:21–28.

6 Vanholder RC, Glorieux GL, De Smet RV: Back to the future: middle molecules, high-flux membranes, and optimal dialysis. Hemodial Int 2003;7:52–57.

7 Hornberger JC, Chernew M, Petersen J, Garber AM: A multivariative analysis of mortality and hospital admission with high-flux dialysis. J Am Soc Nephrol 1992;3:1227–1237.

8 Koda Y, Nishi S, Miyazaki S, et al: Switch from conventional to high-flux membrane reduces the risk of carpal tunnel syndrome and mortality of hemodialysis patients. Kidney Int 1997;52:1096–1101.

9 Hakim RM, Held PJ, Stannard DC, et al: Effect of the dialysis membrane on mortality of chronic hemodialysis patients. Kidney Int 1996;50:566–570.

10 Bloembergen WE, Hakim RM, Stannard DC, et al: Relationship of dialysis membrane and cause-specific mortality. Am J Kidney Dis 1999;33:1–10.

11 Leypoldt JK, Cheung AK, Carroll CE, Stannard DC, Pereira BJG, Agodoa LY, Port FK: Effect of dialysis membranes and middle molecule removal on chronic hemodialysis patient survival. Am J Kidney Dis 1999;33: 349–355.
12 Bonomini V, Coli L, Scolari MP, Stefoni S: Structure of dialysis membranes and long-term clinical outcome. Am J Nephrol 1995; 15:455–462.
13 Locatelli F, Mastrangelo F, Redaelli B, Ronco C, Marcelli D, La Greca G, Orlandini G: Effects of different membranes and dialysis technologies on patient treatment tolerance and nutritional parameters. The Italian Cooperative Dialysis Study Group. Kidney Int 1996;50: 1293–1302.
14 Eknoyan G, Beck GJ, Cheung AK, Daugirdas JT, Greene T, Kusek JW, Allon M, Bailey J, Delmez JA, Depner TA, Dwyer JT, Levey AS, Levin NW, Milford E, Ornt DB, Rocco MV, Schulman G, Schwab SJ, Teehan BP, Toto R, Hemodialysis (HEMO) Study Group: Effect of dialysis dose and membrane flux in maintenance hemodialysis. N Engl J Med 2002; 347:2010–2019.
15 Cheung AK, Levin NW, Greene T, Agodoa L, Bailey J, Beck G, Clark W, Levey AS, Leypoldt JK, Ornt DB, Rocco MV, Schulman G, Schwab S, Teehan B, Eknoyan G: Effects of high-flux hemodialysis on clinical outcomes: results of the HEMO study. J Am Soc Nephrol 2003;14: 3251–3263.
16 Cheung AK, Rocco MV, Yan G, Leypoldt JK, Levin NW, Greene T, Agodoa L, Bailey J, Beck GJ, Clark W, Levey AS, Ornt DB, Schulman G, Schwab S, Teehan B, Eknoyan G: Serum β_2-microglobulin levels predict mortality in dialysis patients: results of the HEMO study. J Am Soc Nephrol 2006; 17:546–555.
17 Locatelli F, Martin-Malo A, Hannedouche T, et al: Effect of membrane permeability on survival of hemodialysis patients. J Am Soc Nephrol 2009;20:645–654.
18 Chauveau P, Nguyen H, Combe C, Chene G, Azar R, Cano N, Canaud B, Fouque D, Laville M, Leverve X, Roth H, Aparicio M, French Study Group for Nutrition in Dialysis: Dialyzer membrane permeability and survival in hemodialysis patients. Am J Kidney Dis 2005;45:565–571.
19 Krane V, Krieter DH, Olschewski M, Marz W, Mann JF, Ritz E, Wanner C: Dialyzer membrane characteristics and outcome of patients with type 2 diabetes on maintenance hemodialysis. Am J Kidney Dis 2007;49: 267–275.
20 Yokoyama H, Kawaguchi T, Wada T, Takahashi Y, Higashi T, Yamazaki S, Fukuhara S, Akiba T, Akizawa T, Asano Y, Kurokawa K, Saito A, J-DOPPS Research Group: Biocompatibility and permeability of dialyzer membranes do not affect anemia, erythropoietin dosage or mortality in Japanese patients on chronic non-reuse hemodialysis: a prospective cohort study from the J-DOPPS II study. Nephron Clin Pract 2008;109:c100–c108.
21 Charra B, Calemard E, Ruffet M, et al: Survival as an index of adequacy of dialysis. Kidney Int 1992;41:1286–1291.
22 Koda Y: Influence of high-flux biocompatible membrane on carpal tunnel syndrome and mortality: author's reply. Am J Kidney Dis 1998;32:338–343.
23 Ward RA: Do clinical outcomes in chronic hemodialysis depend on the choice of a dialyzer? Semin Dial 2011;24:65–71.
24 Masaki T, Gilson J, Leypoldt JK, Cheung AK: Effect of permeability on indices of haemodialysis membrane biocompatibility. Nephrol Dial Transplant 1999;14:1176–1181.
25 Schiffl H: High-flux dialyzers, backfiltration, and dialysis fluid quality. Semin Dial 2011; 24:1–4.
26 Woods HF, Nandakumar M: Improved outcome for haemodialysis patients treated with high-flux membranes. Nephrol Dial Transplant 2000;15(suppl 1):36–42.
27 Tattersall J, Martin-Malo A, Pedrini L, et al: EBPG guideline on dialysis strategies. Nephrol Dial Transplant 2007;22(suppl 2): ii5–ii21.

28 Registry of Japanese Society for Dialysis Therapy (RJSDT): An overview of regular dialysis treatment in Japan as of December 31, 2008. Tokyo, RJSDT, 2009.

29 National Kidney Foundation: K/DOQI clinical practice guidelines and clinical practice recommendations for 2006 updates: hemodialysis adequacy, peritoneal dialysis adequacy and vascular access. Am J Kidney Dis 2006;48(suppl 1):S1–S322.

Yutaka Koda
Koda Medical and Dialysis Clinic
3748 Yoshida, Tsubame, Niigata 959-0264 (Japan)
Tel. +81 256 920 001
E-Mail wg8y-kud@asahi-net.or.jp

Saito A, Kawanishi H, Yamashita AC, Mineshima M (eds): High-Performance Membrane Dialyzers.
Contrib Nephrol. Basel, Karger, 2011, vol 173, pp 70–75

Endotoxin and Bacterial Level of Dialysate Fluid Quality

Yutaka Isakozawa · Shingo Takesawa · Vee David

Department of Medical Engineering, School of Health Science, Kyusyu University of Health and Welfare, Nobeoka, Miyazaki, Japan

Abstract

For dialysis fluid quality criteria, several dialysis centers in Japan have put great effort into keeping endotoxin (ET) levels low, although in many countries the bacterial count measurement for dialysis fluid is widely used. The International Organization for Standardization (ISO) suggests an ET and bacterial level for dialysate fluid quality, and Japan currently also measures the bacterial count. Each country presses forward to revise their domestic criteria based on ISO suggestions. In some Japanese cities, guidelines are currently made for dialysate fluid quality control by referring to ISO values. In many countries it is necessary to push forward these domestic guidelines to hemodialysis centers to keep a low level of ET and bacteria. As one of several actual data, we will describe the ET concentration and bacterial count of dialysis fluid in many Japanese dialysis centers to make clear the relation between ET level and bacterial count.

Evaluation of Dialysate Fluid Quality Using Endotoxin Concentration Measurement

In current hemodialysis therapy, a large pore size membrane to remove low-molecular-weight proteins such as β_2-microglobulin – which will be a causative material of the dialysis amyloidosis – is present in the mainstream for routine treatment. On the other hand, these large pore membranes leak some bacterial contents such as endotoxin (ET) from dialysate to the patient's bloodstream through backfiltration and backdiffusion [1]. It is necessary to avoid these unexpected materials – moving from dialysate to blood – in order to decrease the possibility of serious side effects in hemodialysis patients after long-term treatment over a number of years. ET measurement is commonly performed in almost all

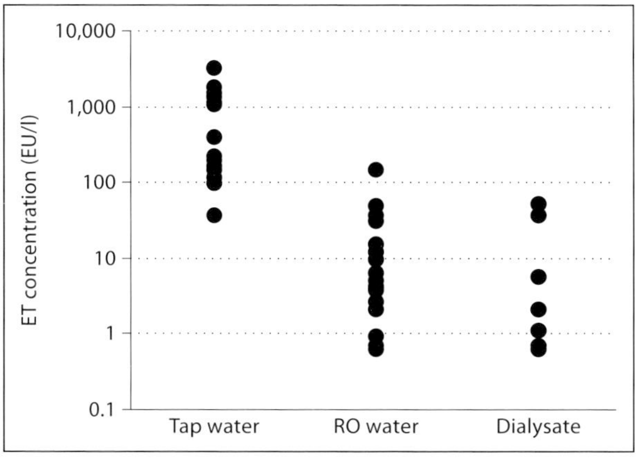

Fig. 1. Dialysate fluid quality survey in Japanese dialysis centers (n = 19).

Japanese dialysis centers. It is a governing reason that the Japanese ET kits must show an extremely high sensitivity, and the measurement result is obtained in a short time. The technologies in these kits make it possible to use them in highly sensitive cases. Only Japanese and some other ET kits show a value of ET concentration of 1 EU/l (= 0.001 EU/ml) precisely as a minimum detection limit. Figure 1 shows the results of a dialysis fluid quality survey in Japanese dialysis centers. The ET levels were as follows: 35–3,134 EU/l in tap water, not detectable to 143 EU/l in reverse osmosis (RO) water, and not detectable to 51 EU/l in dialysate. The average ET concentration was 919 EU/l in tap water, 18 EU/l in RO water, and 6 EU/L in dialysate. These 19 dialysis centers do a relatively higher water control than other centers. There are up to 4,000 dialysis centers in Japan. Figure 1 shows only 2% of the data of Japanese dialysis centers. It is thought that there are many dialysis consoles contaminated with bacteria in Japan.

Dialysate Fluid Quality Evaluation Using the Microbiological Method

The bacterial count measurement for dialysis fluid is widely used in many countries. Some dialysis centers in Japan measure the bacterial count, but it is still uncommon. As for the bacterial count measurement, a membrane filtrate concentration method and a culture by agar plate are taken. The culture method by the flat plate agar is the most basic bacterial count measurement. Reasoner's No. 2 agar (R2A) culture media or tryptone glucose extract agar culture media are suitable for bacterial culture in dialysate. These two culture media were recommended in ISO [2]. There are several advantages in the flat plate agar culture method, namely (1) selective detection of bacteria and (2) the reasonable cost for measurement. On the other hand, the following disadvantages have appeared:

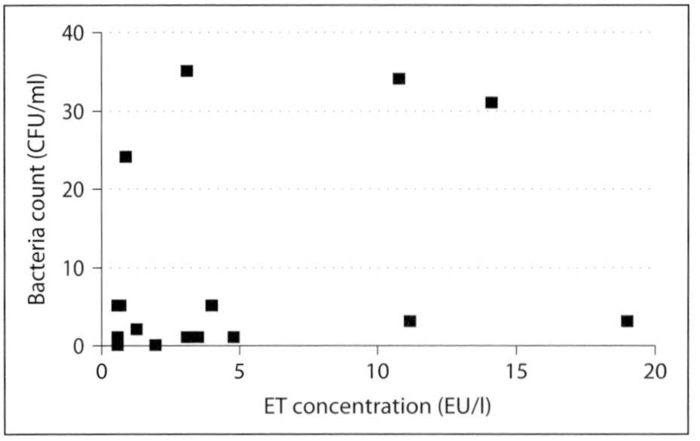

Fig. 2. RO water ET concentration and bacteria count (n = 19, R2A, 2 weeks of culture).

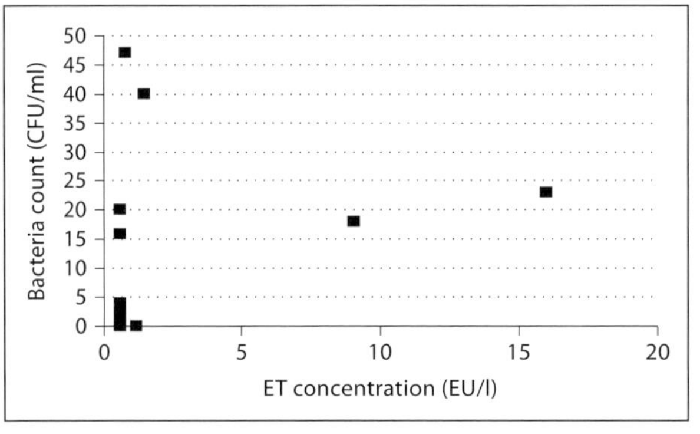

Fig. 3. Dialysate ET concentration and bacteria count (n = 19, R2A, 2 weeks of culture).

(1) only less than 1 ml of sample was available to put on the agar plate, (2) there were many chances for contamination during operation, (3) a very long incubation period is required, and (4) the number of formed colonies was not the same as the number of bacteria. Bacterial count by agar plate was one of the methods for dialysate quality control, but we should remember that the results were not parallel to the number of bacteria in the sample fluid. Figures 2 and 3 show the correlation between ET concentration and bacterial count at 19 dialysis centers. These results were obtained after 2 weeks of culture with R2A media of RO water and dialysate. There were no correlations between ET concentration and bacterial count in these two figures. Especially many bacterial counts were obtained in dialysate fluid of an undetectable level of ET. Ledebo and Nystrand [3] showed that there were no correlations between ET levels and bacterial count, and even if the ET level is less than detectable, bacteria are still present in it. They concluded the need of measuring both ET and bacterial count. The dialysate water quality management criteria of Japan have been revised for these reasons [4, 5].

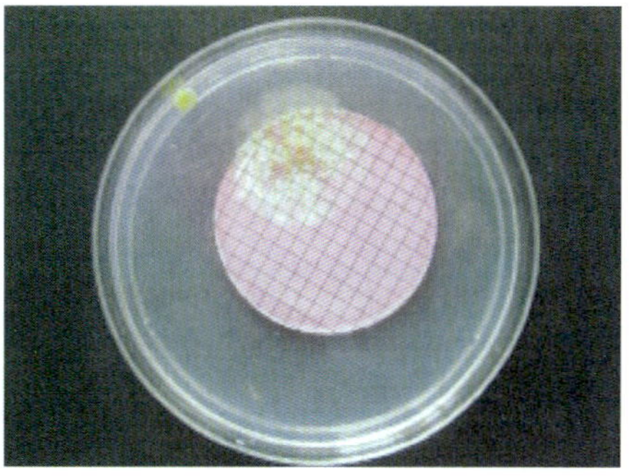

Fig. 4. Contaminated agar plate using the membrane filtrate concentration method.

It is desirable to use a membrane filtrate concentration method in cases with a small number of bacteria. This method can collect bacteria from a large quantity of samples such as 100 ml by filtration, and raise the detectable level of the agar plate culture method. However, using the membrane filtrate concentration method of the open air type, contamination is likely during the filtration process, or during the procedure method. Usually, aseptic processing manipulation is necessary for filtration and removing a membrane filter to the agar plate. Figure 4 shows a case of contamination by the membrane filtrate concentration method. Bacteria and fungi in the environment came into contact with the membrane filter and agar surface, and contamination occurred. Also, we cannot get the colonies unless the filter is completely in contact with the agar plate surface.

In order to decrease the chance of contamination the membrane filtration method of the open air type is impossible at dialysis centers without a clean bench. A 37-mm quality monitor (PALL) and 37-mm monitor (ADVANTEC) were available as the simple membrane filtration method for dialysate fluid quality control. These membrane filters are composed from the cartridge structure with little contaminations. As the operation with a syringe is possible, and liquid culture medium will be injected into a cartridge after the filtration, there is almost no chance of contamination. In many hemodialysis centers, bacterial count evaluation is easily done without a clean bench using this method.

Anti-Biofilm Procedure in Dialysate Fluid Line

The central dialysate delivery system is adopted in almost all Japanese dialysis facilities. It has a very large merit to distribute the same concentration dialysate to many dialysis consoles, but there are also many points for bacterial growth caused by a structure of complicated dialysate piping. It is important that these pipe streams should be simplified as a basic structure for the dialysate fluid line. Dead spaces and connecting parts are one of the hotbeds of biofilms, and these points must be decreased from the dialysate fluid line. Also, it will be necessary

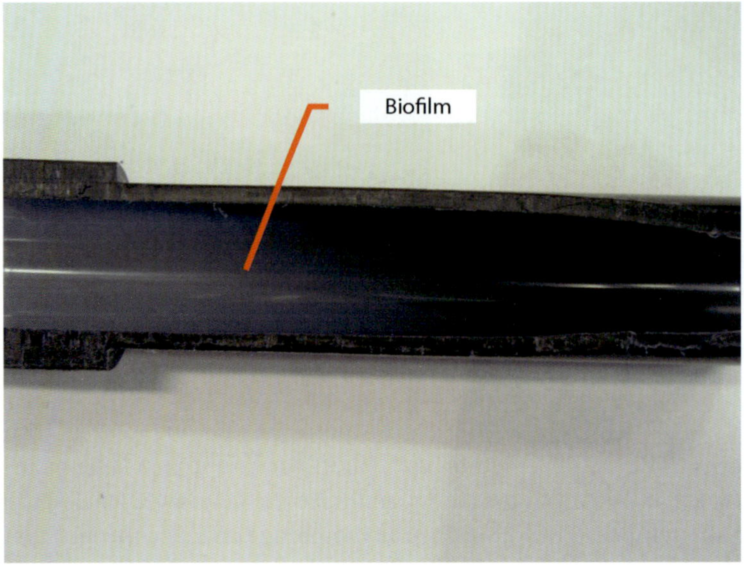

Fig. 5. Biofilm in the PVC pipe for the RO water line.

to fill up the disinfectants in these lines after hemodialysis overnight to keep a low level of bacterial growth. When bacteria grow in biofilms, it is very difficult to remove them by regular disinfectants. The biofilm is an aggregate of bacteria and some other components such as calcium bicarbonate surrounded with the slime of microbe excretes. The main structure is the polysaccharide of bacterial secrete. It is said that most bacteria exist in this biofilm. It is possible to have contact with the biofilm anywhere in the surroundings. For a typical case of biofilm, the plaque in our mouth is a common example. Nominated factors influencing formation of the biofilm are as follows: (1) materials of the pipes or tubes for the dialysate line, (2) total contact area, (3) surface structure, (4) flow rate of dialysate fluid, and (5) microcirculation in connecting parts. The materials of the pipes or tubes slightly influence the formation of the biofilm, and there are no materials for the dialysate line where bacteria cannot contact its surface.

Figure 5 shows an example of the biofilm in a polyvinyl chloride pipe. The white gradation coating on the inside of the pipe is biofilm. This gradation coating is removed mechanically. The study for rejection of the biofilm formation in the dialysis fluid line is inferior. The biofilm is formed not only in pipes or tubes, but also in dialysis devices. Furthermore, it is difficult to fix the appropriate concentrations and temperature of the disinfectant, because of the influence to the pipes or tubes and hemodialysis consoles of high concentration and high temperature of the fluid. It is impossible to maintain perfect sterility. We should suppress bacterial growth, and it is important to know the bacterial count in dialysate fluid of daily use at least once a month.

Conclusion

Dialysate fluid quality has improved dramatically due to wide measurement of ET concentrations in many dialysate centers, and because of data comparison among the centers. Also, in recent years, there were fewer complications in patients on long-term hemodialysis treatment.

Dialysate fluid quality control is involved not only in the improvement of the vital prognosis of patients, but also in quality of life. The bioactivity of ET is said to be increased tens of thousands by coexistence of materials [6]. Unless we do not adopt the correct sampling method, there is no point in measuring the ET concentration and bacterial count in RO dialysate water. To maintain a high-quality control of dialysate fluid, not only the bacterial count measurement by the bacterial agar culture, but also ET concentration measurement is indispensable. When the ET concentration reaches a single value in EU/l or less than the detectable level, we should attempt the bacterial count using the membrane filtration method in order to decrease bacterial content in the dialysate fluid. Furthermore, dialysate line management including biofilm prevention will become a serious problem in the future.

References

1 Pacitti A, Tetta C, Mangiarotti G, et al: Beta-2-microglobulin serum profiles in different settings of mass transport and fluid pyrogen content. Kidney Int Suppl 1993;41:S96–S99.

2 ISO/CD23500: Fluids for haemodialysis and related therapies, 2005.

3 Ledebo I, Nystrand R: Defining the microbiological quality of dialysis fluid. Artif Organs 1999;23:37–43.

4 Kawanishi H, Masakane I, Tomo T: The new standard of fluids for hemodialysis in Japan. Blood Purif 2009;27(suppl 1):5–10.

5 Masakane I, Takemoto Y, Nakai S, et al: Bacteriological water quality in the central dialysis fluid delivery system from the survey of the Japanese Society for Dialysis Therapy. Blood Purif 2009;27(suppl 1):11–16.

6 Rakhmilevich AL, Shneiderova MA, Korobko VG, Chuvpilo SA: Enhancement of tumour necrosis factor production and sensitivity to interleukin-2 of human peripheral blood mononuclear cells stimulated by lipopolysaccharide and muramyl dipeptide in vitro. Biomed Sci 1990;1:517–523.

Yutaka Isakozawa
Department of Medical Engineering, School of Health Science
Kyusyu University of Health and Welfare
1714-1 Yoshinomachi, Nobeoka, Miyazaki 882-8508 (Japan)
Tel. +81 982 235 610, E-Mail isa@phoenix.ac.jp

Saito A, Kawanishi H, Yamashita AC, Mineshima M (eds): High-Performance Membrane Dialyzers.
Contrib Nephrol. Basel, Karger, 2011, vol 173, pp 76–83

Albumin Loss Under the Use of the High-Performance Membrane

Kenji Tsuchida · Jun Minakuchi

Department of Kidney Disease (Artificial Kidney and Kidney Transplantation), Kawashima Hospital, Tokushima City, Tokushima, Japan

Abstract

Beta-2-microglobulin (β_2M) clearance has been improved in recent dialysis membranes and minimum albumin leakage has been achieved in most membranes today since dialysis membranes are now classified by β_2M clearance in terms of the reimbursement by health insurance. Kawanishi et al. suggested that 'the desirable albumin leakage in one treatment is less than 4 g'. Function classification type IV or type V dialysis membranes have leakages as low as 3 g, while most resulted in <1 g leakage. However, some high-performance membranes (HPMs) have around 8 g of leakage, which requires further study of the clinical efficacy using such dialysis membranes. The comparison of albumin leakage in one dialysis treatment (4 h: blood flow volume of 250 ml/min) revealed that PES-210D has an overwhelmingly high albumin leakage of 7.69 ± 1.01 g. The data were without any significant difference between the PES-D membrane user group and the non-PES-D membrane user group for hemoglobin, hematocrit, β_2M protein, catabolic rate, body mass index, and muscle mass. However, the PES-D membrane user group had a significantly lower number of hospitalizations and other complication events. When comparing the event contents, the PES-D membrane user group had no cardiac failure and lower DRA, however it had more vascular access problems. In normal renal function, approximately 10 g of albumin is filtered in the glomerulus per day, decomposed in the renal tubule and reabsorbed as amino acid, and re-synthesized into albumin in the liver. On the contrary, in dialysis patients, albumin that is bound to biologically active substances and/or the oxidized form of albumin that has lost its antioxidant effect cannot be filtered from the kidney and accumulate. Therefore, the idea regarding albumin leakage is to remove biologically active substances that bind to albumin and function as uremic toxin, remove albumin without the antioxidant effect, and facilitate synthesis of new albumin with an antioxidant effect.

It is presumed that the number of substances that accumulate in the body of patients with kidney dysfunction reaches thousands including the products of metabolism of the internal organs. The molecular weight of the substances vary widely from the low to moderate molecular weight region of urea, creatinine, or uric acid, to low-molecular-weight protein represented by β_2-microglobulin (β_2M), or even high-molecular-weight cut-off that covers from globulin to lipid. Pathogenic mechanisms of some of these substances have been proven, such as β_2M in dialysis-related amyloidosis (DRA), however, pathogenic significances in most of the accumulated substances remain to be defined. Safety regarding these substances whose pathogenic significances are not yet clarified also remains to be confirmed. Therefore, under the current circumstances, it is essential to administer a treatment that can get as close to the glomerulus basement membrane as possible, use dialysis membrane to effectively remove a wide range of substances, and aim to remove all of the substances including albumin accumulated in the body of patients with kidney dysfunction.

Development of Protein-Permeable Dialysis Membrane: High-Performance Membrane

In the 1960s, the early years of dialysis therapy, only low-molecular-weight uremic substances such as potassium, urea, creatinine, uric acid, and guanidine compound were removed, which was successful for a limited prolongation of patients' lives.

In 1971, Babb et al. [1] proposed the middle molecule hypothesis, which explains that uremic substances including neurotoxin that causes peripheral nerve disorders exist in the region of middle molecules ranging from a molecular weight of 500 to 5,000. In accordance with the middle molecule hypothesis, the square meter-hour hypothesis was formulated, which assumed that it is membrane area and hours of dialysis, not blood or dialysis fluid flow rates, that determine the efficiency in the removal of middle molecules if using the same dialysis membrane. Following these hypotheses, long-time dialysis using large-size dialysis membrane and the protein-permeable dialysis membrane what we call 'high-performance membrane' (HPM), hemodialysis (HD) methods became more actively implemented based on the ideas that filtration is more effective than dialysis for the removal of middle molecules.

Later in 1985, Gejyo et al. [2] found that the major constituent protein of DRA is β_2M. Since then, β_2M has been considered the target in blood purification therapy and the focus is placed on the development of dialysis membrane with high efficiency of β_2M removal. The sieving coefficient for β_2M was <0.5 at that time as opposed to >0.9 in recent years.

Removal of Uremic Substances and Loss of Albumin in the Low-Molecular-Weight Protein Region and Clinical Efficiency

As mentioned, many cases showed insufficient improvement in the clinical outcome contrary to the decrease in serum β_2M concentration in HD/HDF using HPM with less albumin leakage targeting β_2M, which suggests that the occurrence of clinical symptoms is affected by substances in the larger molecular weight region. Over 2,000 substances have been reported as being uremic substances that are accumulated or produced due to renal failure that causes various clinical symptoms and complications. These substances include many medium- to large-molecular-weight substances such as β_2M. Focusing on these facts, HD/HDF therapy, which associates albumin loss, was implemented targeting the substances in the regions whose molecular weights are larger than β_2M. HD/HDF therapy with HPM, compared to the therapy without HPM, achieved higher success in the removal of larger molecular weight substances including β_2M, cytokine, homocysteine and complement factor D, and higher clinical outcomes were reported, such as prevention of development of DRA, anemia, osteoarthritis and pruritus, and improvement in life prognosis and biocompatibility in Japan.

Albumin Leakage during a Dialysis Treatment

Although albumin usually reflects nutritional status, it is also reported that, in the case of renal insufficiency, albumin is relevant to inflammation or arteriosclerosis as seen in malnutrition inflammation atherosclerosis (MIA) [3] and it affects cardiovascular complication or survival rate. However, β_2M clearance has been improved in recent dialysis membranes and minimum albumin leakage has been achieved in most membranes today since dialysis membranes are now classified by β_2M clearance in terms of the reimbursement by health insurance (table 1) and also because HD membranes are being used for HDF. Among the studies on albumin leakage up to date, Kawanishi et al. [4] suggested that 'the desirable albumin leakage in one treatment is less than 4 g' in their report on the new standard for dialysis fluid quality and functional classification of dialysis membrane.

Albumin Leakage per One Dialysis Treatment for Different HPMs That Have Been on the Market

Figure 1 shows the comparison of the albumin leakage per one dialysis treatment using different HPMs that have been released in Japan. Function classification type IV or type V dialysis membranes have leakages as low as 3 g,

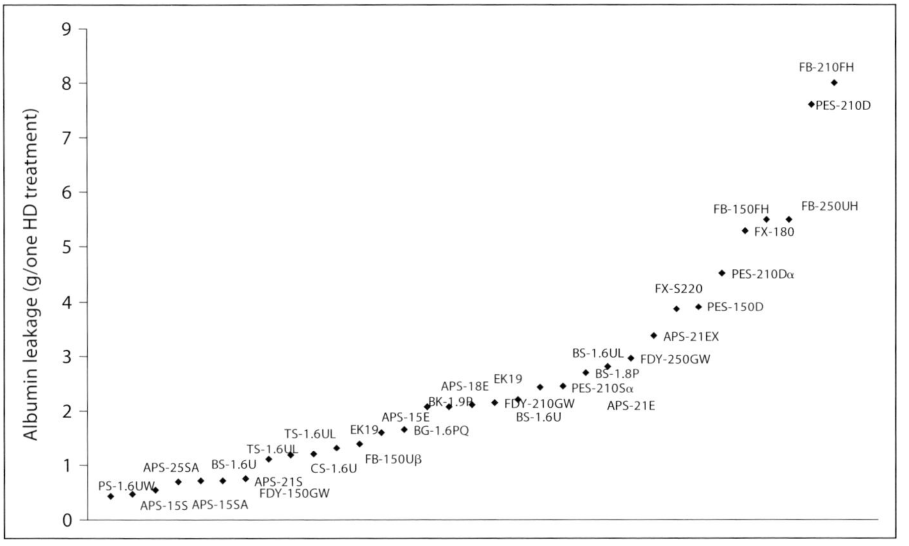

Fig. 1. Albumin leakage per one dialysis treatment for different HPMs.

Table 1. Classification of dialysis membranes in terms of the reimbursement by health insurance in Japan

Classification of dialysis membrane	UFR ml/mm Hg/h	Clearance of urea, ml/min	Clearance of β_2M, ml/min
Type I	3.0⩽	125⩽	
Type II	3.0⩽	150⩽	10⩽ <30
Type III	3.0⩽	150⩽	30⩽ <50
Type IV	3.0⩽	150⩽	50⩽<70
Type V	3.0⩽	150⩽	70⩽

Q_B = 200 ml/min, Q_F = 10 ml/min.

while most resulted in <1 g leakage. However, some HPMs have around 8 g of leakage, which requires further study of the clinical efficacy using such dialysis membranes.

HD Treatment Using PES-D Membrane

The study group that received treatments using the HPM type IV dialysis membrane polyethersulfone (PES)-D series (Nipro) showed a significantly lower

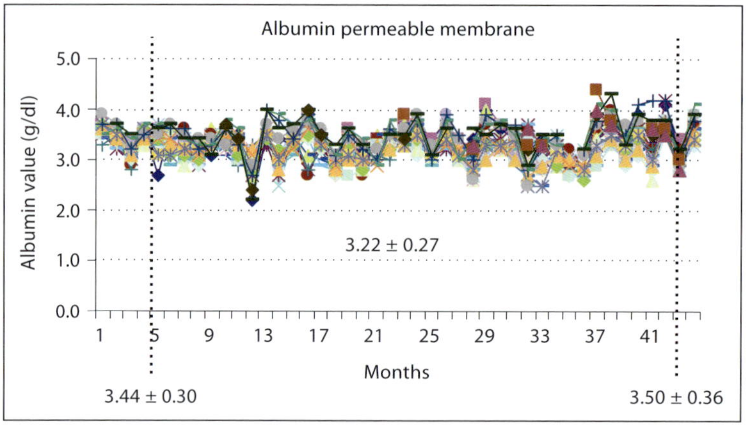

Fig. 2. Effect of the HPM-HD (PES-D) on serum albumin value.

level of serum albumin and total protein and a significantly higher level of total cholesterol. Moreover, the comparison of albumin leakage in one dialysis treatment (4 h: blood flow volume of 250 ml/min) revealed that PES-210D has an overwhelmingly high albumin leakage of 7.69 ± 1.01 g.

Study Using PES-D Membranes

Patients who received HD treatment in the 3-year period from April 2005 to the end of March 2007 were divided into two groups: one received HD treatment with PES-D membrane (n = 118) and the other without PES-D membrane (n = 314) to conduct retrospective studies on the following: (1) monthly shift in serum albumin volume before/after using the PES-D membrane; (2) comparison of various biochemical data or other membranes (average value from six times of comparison held every April and October), and (3) comparison of hospitalization and other complication events.

The results for the points 1 to 3 above were as follows:

(1) Regarding the shift in serum albumin volume before/after the use of membranes, the average albumin concentration measured 3 months before the use of PES-D membrane was 3.44 ± 0.30 g/dl, but the albumin started decreasing 1 month after using PES-D and resulted in the monthly average of albumin concentration of 3.22 ± 0.27 g/dl during the 3 years of treatment using PES-D membrane. In addition, albumin increased 1 month after changing to non-PES-D membrane and the average albumin concentration in 3 months after the change was 3.50 ± 0.36 g/dl (fig. 2).

(2) In the comparison of various biochemical data of other membranes, there were no significant differences in hemoglobin as it was 10.9 ± 1.14 g/dl for the

PES-D membrane user group and 10.8 ± 1.21 g/dl for the non-PES-D membrane user group. The following values in parentheses indicate PES-D membrane user group vs. non-PES-D membrane user group, significant difference. The data without any significant difference between the two groups were: hematocrit (32.7 ± 3.76 vs. 32.4 ± 3.80%, n.s.), β_2M (27.9 ± 7.12 vs. 27.4 ± 5.98 g/l, n.s.), protein catabolic rate (1.00 ± 0.18 vs. 1.00 ± 0.20 g/day, n.s.), body mass index (21.3 ± 2.66 vs. 22.0 ± 3.60 kg/m^2, n.s.), muscle mass (43.3 ± 9.73 vs. 43.5 ± 7.90 kg, n.s.), age (64.2 ± 13.6 vs. 63.8 ± 12.0 years old, n.s.), and history of dialysis (10.1 ± 6.1 vs. 11.7 ± 2.3 year, n.s.). The data that proved to be significantly low values for the PES-D user group were: serum total protein concentration (6.28 ± 0.52 vs. 6.35 ± 0.47 g/dl, $p < 0.0005$) and serum albumin concentration (3.52 ± 0.39 vs. 3.63 ± 0.35 g/dl, $p < 0.0001$).

(3) In the comparison of hospitalization and other complication events, the PES-D membrane user group had a significantly lower number of hospitalizations and other complication events. When comparing the event contents, the PES-D membrane user group had no cardiac failure and lower DRA, however it had more vascular access problems (fig. 3a, b).

Human Mercaptalbumin and Non-Mercaptalbumin

Studies suggest that albumin absorbs albumin binding toxin and various uremic substances [5]. It is inferable that the dialysis membrane with higher albumin leakage would also have leakage of amino acid or other necessary proteins, however, as far as dialysis treatment is concerned, the accumulation of uremic substances is more of a problem than albumin leakage. According to the report studying the ratio of non-mercaptalbumin (oxidized albumin) and human mercaptalbumin (reduced albumin) in various HPMs, the group using HPM with higher albumin leakage has more reduced albumin in the body [6]. Although the half-life period for albumin is known to be around 20 days, it is assumed that the metabolism will be boosted for the emergence of albumin and the reduction reserve for active oxygen will be recovered by actively removing the albumin damaged by uremic substances.

Conclusion

The primary idea regarding albumin leakage in dialysis therapy is that a certain level of albumin leakage cannot be avoided in order to increase the volume of the removal of low-molecular-weight substances and low molecular protein that are accumulated in blood. Locatelli et al. [7] reported on the effect of membrane permeability on survival of HD patients. It was reported that a significant survival benefit with either high- or low-flux membranes in the population overall,

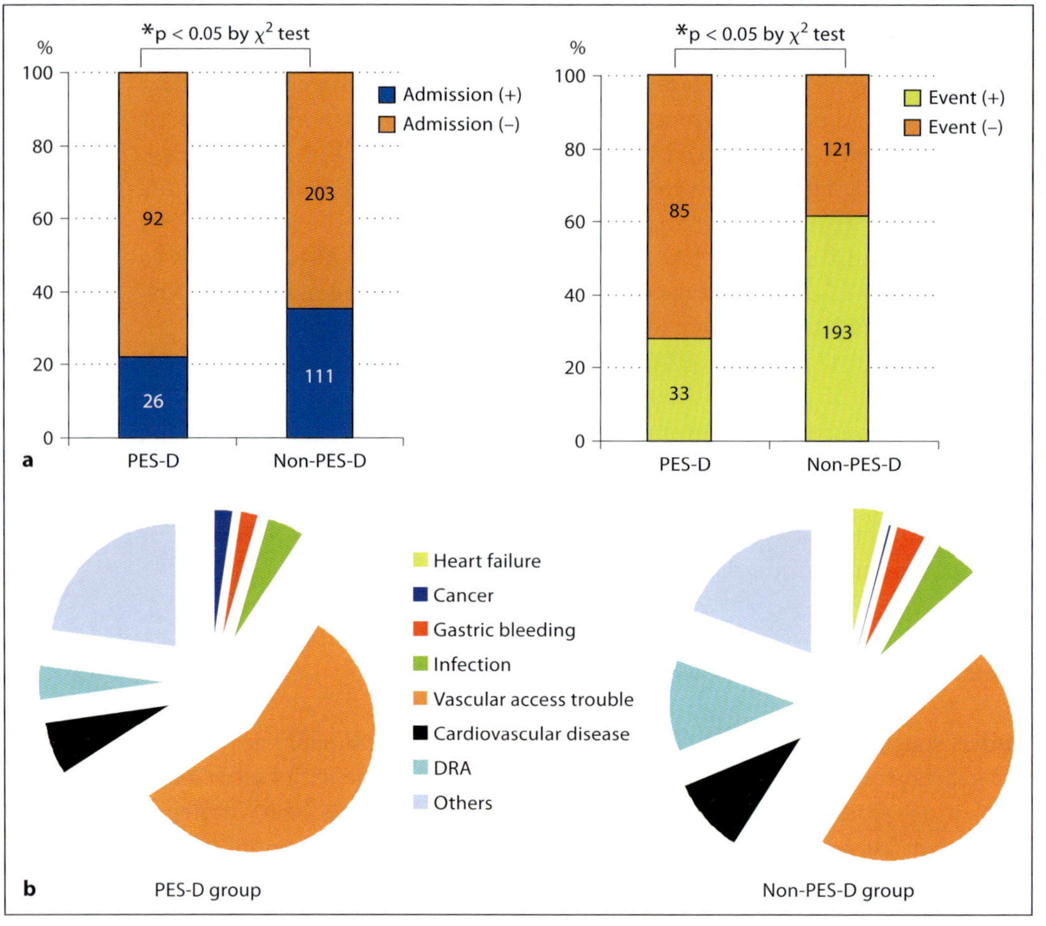

Fig. 3. Effect of the PES-D membrane user group on the (**a**) frequencies of hospitalization and (**b**) occurrence of complications.

but the use of high-flux membranes conferred a significant survival benefit among patients with serum albumin ≤4 g/dl. The apparent survival benefit among patients who have diabetes and are treated with high-flux membranes requires confirmation given the post-hoc nature of our analysis. Meanwhile, albumin has various roles in the body such as maintaining colloid osmotic pressure, transportation and absorption of hormone, fatty acid, medical substances and other biologically active substances, pH buffer action and antioxidant action. In normal renal function, approximately 10 g of albumin is filtered in the glomerulus per day, decomposed in the renal tubule and reabsorbed as amino acid, and re-synthesized into albumin in the liver. On the contrary, in dialysis patients, albumin that is bound to biologically active substances and/or the oxidized form of albumin that has lost its antioxidant effect cannot be filtered from the kidney and accumulate. Therefore, the second idea regarding albumin leakage is to remove biologically active substances that bind to albumin and function as uremic toxin, remove albumin without the antioxidant effect, and facilitate synthesis of new albumin with an antioxidant effect. Acceleration of albumin metabolism not only helps the removal of uremic toxic substances, but also the maintenance of albumin functions.

References

1 Babb AL, Popovich RP, Christopher TG, Scribner BH: The genesis of the square meter-hour hypothesis. Trans Am Soc Artif Intern Organs 1971;17:81–91.

2 Gejyo F, Yamada T, Odani S, Nakagawa Y, Arakawa M, Kunitomo T, Kataoka H, Suzuki M, Hirasawa Y, Shirahama T, et al: A new form of amyloid protein associated with chronic hemodialysis was identified as β_2-microglobulin. Biochem Biophys Res Commun 1985;129:701–706.

3 Stenvinkel P, Heimburger O, Paultre F, et al. Strong associations between malnutrition, inflammation and atherosclerosis in chronic renal failure. Kidney Int 1999;55:1899–1911.

4 Kawanishi H, Mineshima M, Takesawa S, Masakane I, Minakuchi J, Akisawa T, Saito A: New standard of dialysis fluid and classification of dialysis membrane. 2005;38:149–154.

5 Niwa T: Update of uremic toxin research by mass spectrometry. Mass Spectrom Rev 2011;30:510–521.

6 Terawaki H, Yoshimura K, Hasegawa T, Matsuyama Y, Negawa T, Yamada K, Matsushima M, Nakayama M, Hosoya T, Era S: Oxidative stress is enhanced in correlation with renal dysfunction: examination with the redox state of albumin. Kidney Int 2004;66: 1988–1993.

7 Locatelli F, Martin-Malo A, Hannedouche T, Loureiro A, Papadimitriou, M, Wizemann V, Jacobson SH, Czekalski S, Ronco C, Vanholder R: Membrane Permeability Outcome (MPO) Study Group: Effect of membrane permeability on survival of hemodialysis patients. J Am Soc Nephrol 2009;20:645–654.

Kenji Tsuchida
Department of Kidney Disease, Kawashima Hospital
1-39 Kita-sako, Ichiban-cho
Tokushima City, Tokushima 770-8548 (Japan)
Tel. +81 88 631 0110, E-Mail ktsuchida@khg.or.jp

Saito A, Kawanishi H, Yamashita AC, Mineshima M (eds): High-Performance Membrane Dialyzers.
Contrib Nephrol. Basel, Karger, 2011, vol 173, pp 84–94

Choice of Modality with the Use of High-Performance Membrane and Evaluation for Clinical Effects

Ikuto Masakane

Yabuki Shima Clinic, Yamagata, Japan

Abstract

The golden target for dialysis therapy should be to guarantee longer survival and to give a higher quality of life without dialysis-related complications. In order to achieve this target, the choice of dialysis modality and membrane is essential but we have not yet established what the best choice for a dialysis modality and membrane are. Generally, we choose a dialysis modality for better solute removal and better biocompatibility. In this issue we would like to propose that the patients' preference for dialysis therapy is a useful parameter in prescribing the dialysis modality. In our recent experience, chronic dialysis patients have had preferences on a dialysis modality and membrane, those being PMMA, EVAL, AN-69 and pre-dilution online HDF. These modalities could relieve them of uncomfortable dialysis-related symptoms such as insomnia, itchiness, irritability, and so on. Other characteristics of these modalities are of a nutritional advantage, a broad removal pattern of uremic toxins including low-molecular-weight protein and protein-bound uremic toxins, and good biocompatibility free from chemical components of dialysis membrane. In conclusion, patients' symptoms could be a useful parameter to choose a dialysis modality and membrane.

'High-performance membrane' (HPM) is a unique term originally coined in Japan in the early 1980s and has still only been used inside Japan. It is similar to but not the same as the term 'high-flux membrane', which has been widely used throughout the world. The concept of HPM is composed of high water permeability, high permeability in solute removal, high protein-leaking property, better biocompatibility and other possible beneficial effects to the dialysis patient. Many membranes composed of various materials and permeability have been developed in the world. Recently, one of most interest related to HPM is how to prescribe dialysis modality with HPM and how to choose a membrane from enormous line-ups of HPM.

Generally we choose a dialysis membrane based on a better solute removal property, but there has been no evidence that has proven that membranes with a higher permeability always have a better outcome. If we use the same dialysis membrane for hemodialysis (HD) and hemodiafiltration (HDF), each solute removal pattern would not be the same and would result in a different outcome. Therefore, we have not established a strategy on how to choose a dialysis modality or dialysis membrane for the sake of a good clinical outcome. In this article we would like to propose guidance on how to make this important decision.

Dialysis Modality and the Latest Trend in Japan

The Japanese Society for Dialysis Therapy (JSDT) has surveyed the status of dialysis therapy as of the 31st of December annually since 1968. From the 2008 JSDT database, 282,622 patients were on chronic dialysis [1]. 273,276 patients (96.7%) were treated by center dialysis, 9,157 patients (3.2%) were on peritoneal dialysis, and only 194 (0.1%) patients were on home HD. Center dialysis included HD (93.3%), HDF (6.6%), and hemofiltration (0.1%). Various types of HDF had been performed; bottle-type HDF (offline HDF) was used for 57.5% of the HDF patients, online HDF was used for 38.3%, acetate-free biofiltration was used for 2.7% and push/pull HDF was used for 1.5%. β_2-Microglobulin (β_2MG) adsorbent column (Lixelle®) was used for 0.6% of the center dialysis patients [1].

All dialyzers in Japan have been classified into seven categories based on their clearance of β_2MG (Cl-β_2MG) and other characters since 2006 and each dialyzer has been reimbursed in a different price. The categories are: type 1: Cl-β_2MG (ml/min) <10; type 2: 10 = <Cl-β_2MG (ml/min) <30; type 3: 30 = <Cl-β_2MG (ml/min) <50; type 4: 50 = <Cl-β_2MG (ml/min) <70; type 5: 70 = <Cl-β_2MG (ml/min); type 6: 'hemodiafilter', which is officially permitted for use in HDF, and its Cl-β_2MG is usually >50, and type 7: flat plate type (most of which is made of AN-69).

From the 2008 JSDT survey, prevalence of each category was 1.3, 1.0, 4.2, 80.3, 11.4, 0.2, and 1.2% respectively in HD, and 0.2, 0.2, 2.0, 59.8,16.3, 18.8, and 1.6% in HDF. The membrane materials were polysulfone (PS) as 52.7%, polyethersulfone (PES) as 11.3%, polyethersulfone polymer alloy (PEPA) as 7.6%, polymethylmethacrylate (PMMA) as 5.1%, modified cellulosics as 19.4%, and others. In accordance to the data, more than 90% of patients were treated by synthetic membrane such as PS and PES with marked high permeability in Japan. When we use high permeable membranes for HD or HDF, we should keep the biological water quality as clean as possible. The water quality in most Japanese dialysis facilities has been proven to meet the JSDT standard for using high permeable membranes [2].

General Concept for Choosing a Dialysis Modality and Membrane Material

A golden target for dialysis therapy should be to guarantee a longer survival and to give a higher quality of life without dialysis-related complications. We wanted to choose a dialysis modality and dialysis membrane in order to achieve this target based on evidence, however we have little evidence that has proven the effectiveness of some dialysis modalities and dialysis membranes on patient survival. Canaud et al. [3] reported that only high-efficiency (online) HDF had an advantage on patient survival compared to low- or high-efficiency HD and low-efficiency HDF. This study was performed as a prospective cohort study, however the patient selection bias and other problems concerning the study design have been pointed out. Several randomized control prospective studies have failed to prove a distinct advantage of high-flux membrane on patient survival [4, 5], so we have not yet had reliable evidence for choosing a dialysis modality and membrane.

HPM was originally developed in order to eliminate middle molecular substances which were previously unable to be eliminated by cellulosic membrane. After β_2MG was identified as a precursor to dialysis-related amyloidosis (DRA) fibril in 1985, the main purpose of the use of HPM had become to eliminate β_2MG effectively for the protection of DRA. β_2MG is an important low-molecular-weight protein (LMWP) not only as an essential element of DRA, but as an indicator of patient survival and a parameter for evaluating the performance of the dialysis membrane. The serum level of β_2MG has been recognized as an independent prognostic factor for chronic dialysis patients. The lower level of β_2MG than around 30 mg/l has been reported to be favorable for good patient survival [6], but it has still been controversial whether or not more β_2MG removal could result in longer patient survival. The serum level of β_2MG is affected by many factors, such as residual renal function, the removal efficacy in dialysis, inflammatory status of the patient, and so on.

Biocompatibility of dialysis therapy is another important issue for choosing a dialysis modality and membrane. Various types of synthetic dialysis membranes have been developed to improve the bioincompatibility which was seen in the original cellulosic membrane. Bioincompatibility in dialysis therapy has been recognized as an important pathogen of dialysis-related complications such as DRA and malnutrition. Dialysis membrane is usually centered on the property of solute removal but it is rarely concerned with a dialysis prescription for each individual patient.

The last indispensable factor for choosing dialysis modality is the medical reimbursement system in each country. In Japan, officially permitted clinical indications on HDF were DRA and intradialytic hypotension. Furthermore, online HDF had not been officially permitted before 2010. Although online HDF requires more additional costs for keeping the dialysis water quality ultrapure, the total reimbursed cost for online HDF is lower than that for

HD. These socio-economical limitations in the medical reimbursement system have been the main factor inhibiting the progression of online HDF utilization.

New Concept for Choosing a Dialysis Modality and Membrane Material

Body mass has been recognized as one of the most powerful predictors for patient survival in dialysis patients [7]. In dialysis patients, uremic retentive solutes and bioincompatibility of the dialysis therapy itself have been known to lead to microinflammation, and it would be a common pathogenesis of various dialysis-related complications [8]. Malnutrition inflammation atherosclerosis (MIA) syndrome is the most important issue among these complications [9]. If we made a dialysis prescription based on that which could sustain body mass, it could be useful in choosing a dialysis modality and membrane.

Chronic dialysis patients frequently complain about itchiness, irritability, depression, disturbed sleep and other dialysis-related symptoms. Some of these symptoms have been known as significant predictors for patient mortality [10, 11]. If we could make a dialysis prescription to ameliorate these symptoms, it must be a good guide to choose a dialysis modality. In our recent experiences, many patients in our facilities have preferred dialyzers made of PMMA, ethylene vinyl alcohol copolymer (EVAL), AN-69 or pre-dilution online HDF mode [12]. We found that these dialysis modalities could relieve their dialysis-related symptoms and sustain muscle volume [12]. In other words, patient preference could also be a new parameter for choosing a dialysis modality or a membrane. We named this therapeutic concept the 'patient-oriented dialysis system' – the POD system [12].

Results of the Dialysis Prescription Based on the POD System

We have two basic questionnaires given in our POD system and we perform them twice a year. The POD sheet has 36 questions regarding the quality of their life and the symptoms experienced related to their dialysis. The malnutrition inflammation score (MIS) sheet is an assessment tool used for the screening of the nutritional status originally created by Kalantar-Zadeh et al. [13]. If the patients have any problems in the POD sheet and MIS sheet, dialysis therapies and nutritional approaches will be reconsidered and changed in order to solve the problems. In this therapeutic concept, the choice of a dialysis membrane and online HDF are major keys for achieving a good dialysis. Over 90% of our patients have been treated by EVAL, PMMA, AN-69 membranes, pre-dilution online HDF mode, and especially EVAL was used in all newly starting dialysis patients (fig. 1).

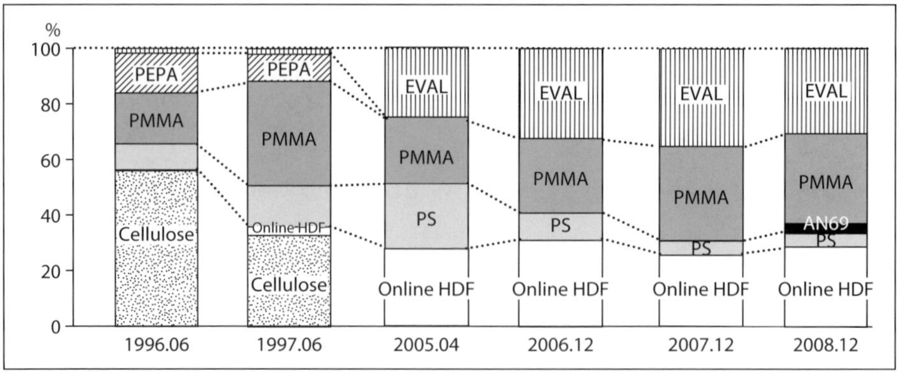

Fig. 1. Changes in the selection of dialysis membranes (in HD mode) or HDF mode (with PS membrane) in our facilities. Recently the majority have been PMMA, EVAL and online HDF.

Uremic pruritus is one of the most frequent symptoms we confront and has been recognized to be associated with a higher mortality risk and sleep disturbance. The prevalence of more than moderate itching was reported to be relatively high, 40–50%, but only 15% of patients complained about itchiness in our facilities [10, 12]. The prevalence of sleep disturbance as 'poor' or 'bad' was 18% and it was less frequent than that of DOPPS by one third [12].

In order to evaluate the advantage of the POD system, a 5-year-survival rate in our facilities was compared with that of JSDT. The accumulated 5-year survival rate was 77% in our facilities and 57% in JSDT, although the mean age of the patients was 69 years and was 3 years older than that of JSDT [12]. The 5-year-survival rate of the older patients was 52% in our facilities and 27% in JSDT. The POD system enables chronic dialysis patients to live longer without uncomfortable dialysis-related symptoms.

Rationale of the POD System

Solute Removal Pattern and Nutritional Advantage

In the preliminary study, we found that pre-dilution online HDF could maintain the muscle volume of the dialysis patients [12]. In order to clarify why pre-dilution HDF has a nutritional advantage, we compared the solute removal pattern between HD, pre-dilution online HDF, and post-dilution online HDF. Small solute removal was reduced but amino acids were better preserved in pre-dilution online HDF than in HD or post-dilution HDF. On the other hand, LMWPs such as β_2MG (MW 12 kDa) or leptin (MW 16 kDa) were effectively removed in HDF, especially in the pre-dilution HDF mode of our therapeutic prescription [12]. Albumin loss per session was 0.8 g in HD, 1.3 g in pre-dilution

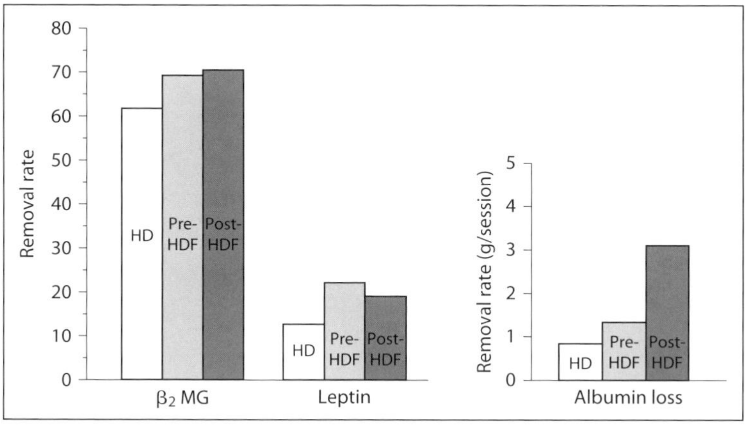

Fig. 2. Removal rates of β_2MG and leptin, and albumin loss. Pre-dilution HDF mode has higher removability of β_2MG or leptin than HD mode, and less albumin loss than post-dilution HDF mode.

HDF, and 3.1 g in post-dilution HDF (fig. 2). The same effect on maintaining body mass has been reported in HD by EVAL, PMMA and AN-69. Muta et al. [14] reported that body mass reduction observed in HD with the PS membrane dramatically improved with the change of the dialysis membrane to EVAL in older dialysis patients. Their hypothesis for the advantage of the EVAL membrane was that the loss of amino acids during a dialysis session was milder in HD with EVAL membrane.

Several recent studies have shown protein-leaking HD or HDF was effective in removing some protein-bound uremic toxins. One of the most typical protein-bound solutes is P-cresol, and it was effectively removed by pre-dilution online HDF rather than HD and post-dilution HDF [15]. Leptin is a well-known uremic toxin which deteriorates the appetite of dialysis patients and has been classified into both of the two uremic toxin groups: protein-bound solute toxins and middle molecules [16]. In our studies, leptin was better removed in pre-dilution online HDF than HD and post-dilution HDF. We supposed that excessive plasma dilution in pre-dilution was an important factor for enhancing the efficacy of the removal of protein-bound uremic toxins. Protein-leaking membranes have been reported to have advantages in removing some LMWP and protein-bound uremic toxins [17].

LMWPs or some albumins are effectively removed by convection in HDF, large pore size in EVAL membrane, or protein adsorptive property in PMMA or PAN membrane. This broad removal pattern of dialysis membranes or pre-dilution online HDF mode might be similar to the native kidneys and have an advantage in keeping body mass in dialysis patients.

Table 1. Bisphenol-A and PVP included in dialyzers in Japan (some dialyzers have neither bisphenol-A nor PVP)

Manufacturer	Dialyzer	Membrane material	Housing material	Bisphenol-A		PVP
				membrane	housing	
AsahiKasei-Kuraray	APS-MD, S, E	PS	polystyrene	+	–	+
	PAN-SF	PAN	polystyrene	–	–	–
	KF, KF-C	EVAL	polycarbonate	–	+	–
Toray	TS-UL, PL	PS	polycarbonate	+	+	+[1]
	CS-U	PS	polypropylene	+	–	+[1]
	BK, BG	PMMA	polystyrene	–	–	–
Kawasumi	PS-N, H, UW	PS	polycarbonate	+	+	+
Fresenius	FPX	PS	polycarbonate	+	–	+
Nipro	FB-U, F	CTA	polycarbonate	–	+	–
	PES-D, DS, DE	PES	polycarbonate	–	+	+
Nikkiso	FDY, FDX	PEPA	polycarbonate	+	+	+
Gambro	H12-4000S	PAN	ABS	–	–	–

[1] Cross-linked PVP exists in Toray PS membranes.

Biocompatibility of Dialyzers

Polyvinylpyrrolidone (PVP) is a chemical agent which gives hydrophilicity to hydrophobic products so it is widely used to make many products, such as beverages, soft contact lenses and many synthetic dialysis membranes. PVP is an indispensable component to make PS, PES and many other synthetic membranes. Bisphenol-A is an essential element used in making plastics and polycarbonate, which is widely used for the dialyzer housing material. However, bisphenol-A is also well known as an environmental hormone or endocrine disrupter. PS is the most widely used membrane material throughout the world but some recent studies have suggested that PS has some uncomfortable side effects such as anaphylaxis, skin lesions and thrombocytopenia, which are supposed to be caused by PVP. There are many dialysis membranes which contain PVP or bisphenol-A, but some membranes do not have them (table 1). In pre-dilution HDF the blood is much more diluted before the dialyzer, and a large amount of fluid is filtered from the blood side to the dialysis fluid side. If the elution of PVP or other chemical components from dialyzer occur, a large amount of fluid could wash these substances out to the dialysis fluid side. Much diluted blood in pre-dilution HDF would enable the reduction of a close contact between blood cells and the dialysis membrane. Shear stress for blood cells would also be milder in pre-dilution than post-dilution, so we could decide that the pre-dilution online HDF is more biocompatible than HD and post-dilution HDF. As we previously mentioned, our patients choose the therapies with PMMA, EVAL, AN-69 membranes and pre-dilution online HDF surely without the knowledge about the nutritional advantages and the chemical components of membranes of these modalities.

Strategies for Choosing a Dialysis Modality and Membrane

A 60-year-old man started to receive maintenance HD using EVAL membrane on March 2004. One year after the initiation when he realized his daily urine volume was almost zero, he had been suffering from irritability. Super high-flux PS membrane (APS-18E) was adopted and the 4-hour dialysis time was extended to 5 h. After a 2-year stable period he had had severe irritability and insomnia, so pre-dilution HDF was provided to relieve the symptoms. Three months after the prescription change, skin pigmentation, eruption and severe itching had worsened. More protein-leaking membrane (FDY-210GW) was used as pre-dilution HDF mode, and then he had had a symptom-free state which lasted for 10 months. In February 2008, he had suffered from uncomfortable abdominal muscle cramps, irritability, and then he had severe insomnia. Home HD was not able to be indicated for him because of his familial problem, so we tried daily center dialysis with protein-leaking high-flux EVAL membrane. After six 4-hour dialysis sessions, his uncomfortable symptoms completely disappeared. Since then he has continued strong protein-leaking modality by PES-21Dα in post-dilution HDF, and dialysis time was 6 h, and another 4-hour session was added biweekly. We have adjusted the filtration flow rate as 30–50 ml/min according his symptoms and the level of serum albumin (table 2).

To summarize, what we have proposed in this issue is how to choose a dialysis modality and membrane material, shown as an algorithm in figure 3. We start a dialysis therapy for all patients with EVAL membrane which has a nice balance of solute removal and protein-leaking property as previously addressed. When the residual renal function disappears or some uremic symptoms occur, we will change a membrane to PMMA, AN-69 and vitamin-E-coated PS. If the symptoms were severe even in the early phase just after the introduction of RRT, we perform pre-dilution online HDF. In both HD and HDF mode, we regulate the protein loss by changing dialysis membrane depending on the symptoms and the level of serum albumin. We usually perform HDF by PS, PEPA, PES in both pre- and post-dilution, and PMMA and AN-69 in post-dilution. When

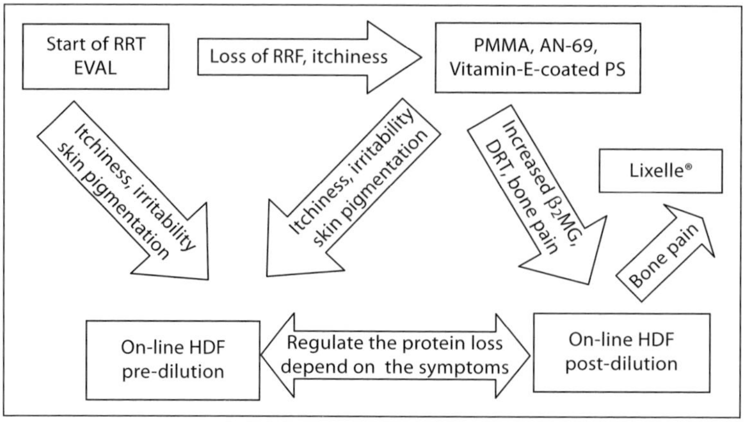

Fig. 3. Algorithm in choosing a dialysis modality and membrane.

Table 2. Example case for prescribing dialysis modalities

Date	Event or symptom	Dialysis prescription
2004.03	starting dialysis	KF12, Q_B 250 ml/min, DT 4 h
2005.01	loss of RRF, irritability	APS-18E, Q_B 250 ml/min, DT 5 h
2007.01	severe irritability, insomnia	APS-18E pre-dilution HDF, Q_B 300 ml/min, Q_F 200 ml/min, DT 5 h
2007.04	pigmentation, skin eruption, severe itching	FDY-210GW pre-dilution HDF, Q_B 300 ml/min, Q_F 200 ml/min, DT 5 h
2008.02	muscle cramp, irritability, insomnia	EK16 daily HD, DT 4 h 6 times/week
2008.08	symptom-free	PES-21Dα, post-dilution HDF, Q_B 300 ml/min, Q_F 50 ml/min, DT 6 h 3 times per week, additional 4 h per 2 weeks
	according to the symptoms	Q_F 30–50 ml/min

bone and joint pain are severe in DRA patients, we add the β_2MG adsorptive column Lixelle®.

Conclusion

The golden target of chronic dialysis should be to guarantee longer survival and to give a higher quality of life in dialysis patients. To achieve this target, it is very important to choose a dialysis modality and a membrane. The important points in choosing a modality are focusing their symptoms and nutritional status. Our patients have preferences for their dialysis treatments such as PMMA, EVAL, AN-69 membranes and pre-dilution online HDF. Our experiences have revealed that these prescriptions ameliorate the various symptoms, nutritional status and survival rate in the dialysis patients. Biocompatibility free from chemical components of dialysis membrane and a well-balanced broad removal pattern of uremic toxins are an essential scientific basis in the patients' preference. In conclusion, patients' symptoms could be a useful parameter to choose a dialysis modality and membrane.

References

1 Tsubakihara Y: An overview of regular dialysis treatment in Japan as of December 31, 2008 (CD-ROM). Tokyo, Japanese Society for Dialysis Therapy, 2009.

2 Masakane I, Tsubakihara Y, Akiba T, et al: Bacteriological qualities of dialysis fluid in Japan as of 31 December 2006. Ther Apher Dial 2008;12:454–460.

3 Canaud B, Morena M, Leray-Moragues H, Chalabi L, Cristol JP: Overview of clinical studies in hemodiafiltration: what do we need now? Hemodial Int 2006;10(suppl 1): S5–S12.

4 Eknoyan G, Beck GJ, Cheung AK, Daugirdas JT, Greene T, Kusek JW, Allon M, Bailey J, Delmez JA, Depner TA, Dwyer JT, Levey AS, Levin NW, Milford E, Ornt DB, Rocco MV, Schulman G, Schwab SJ, Teehan BP, Toto R: Effect of dialysis dose and membrane flux in maintenance hemodialysis. N Engl J Med 2002;347:2010–2019.

5 Locatelli F, Martin-Malo A, Hannedouche T, Loureiro A, Papadimitriou M, Wizemann V, Jacobson SH, Czekalski S, Ronco C, Vanholder R: Effect of membrane permeability on survival of hemodialysis patients. J Am Soc Nephrol 2009;20:645–654.

6 Okuno S, Ishimura E, Kohno K, et al: Serum β_2-microglobulin level is a significant predictor of mortality in maintenance haemodialysis patients. Nephrol Dial Transplant 2009; 24:571–577.

7 Kopple JD, Zhu X, Lew NL, Lowrie EG: Body weight-for-height relationships predict mortality in maintenance hemodialysis patients. Kidney Int 1999;56:1136–1148.

8 Colton CK, Ward RA, Shaldon S: Scientific basis for assessment of biocompatibility in extracorporeal blood treatment. Nephrol Dial Transplant 1994;9(suppl 2):11–17.

9 Stenvinkel P, Heimburger O, Paultre F, Diczfalusy U, Wang T, Berglund L, Jogestrand T: Strong association between malnutrition, inflammation, and atherosclerosis in chronic renal failure. Kidney Int 1999;55:1899–1911.

10 Pisoni R, Wirkstoem B, Elder SJ, Akizawa T, Asano Y, Keen ML, Saran R, Mendelssohn DC, Young EW, Port FK: Pruritus in haemodialysis patients: international results from the Dialysis Outcomes and Practice Patterns Study (DOPPS). Nephrol Dial Transplant 2006;21:3495–3505.

11 Lopes AA, Albert JM, Young EW, Satayathum S, Pisoni RL, Andreucci VE, Mapes DL, Mason NA, Fukuhara S, Wikstrom B, Saito A, Port FK. Screening for depression in hemodialysis patients: associations with diagnosis, treatment, and outcomes in the DOPPS. Kidney Int 2004;66: 2047–2053.

12 Masakane I: High-quality dialysis: a lesson from the Japanese experience. Nephrol Dial Transplant Plus 2010;3(suppl 1):i28–i35.

13 Kalantar-Zadeh K, Kopple JD, Block G, Humphreys MH: A malnutrition-inflammation score is correlated with morbidity and mortality in maintenance hemodialysis patients. Am J Kidney Dis 2001;38:1251–1263.

14 Muta T, Fujimoto T, Harada Y, et al: Are there any differences on amino acid loss during dialysis session by the dialysis membrane material? (in Japanese) Kidney Dial 2005;59(suppl):High Performance Membrane, pp 241–244.
15 Bammens B, Evenepoel P, Verbeke K, Vanrenterghem Y: Removal of the protein-bound solute P-cresol by convective transport: a randomized crossover study. Am J Kidney Dis 2004;44:278–285.
16 Vanholder R, De Smet R, Glorieux G, Argiles A, Baurmeister U, Brunet P, Clark W, Cohen G, De Deyn PP, Deppisch R, Descamps-Latscha B, Henle T, Jorres A, Lemke HD, Massy ZA, Passlick-Deetjen J, Rodriguez M, Stegmayr B, Stenvinkel P, Tetta C, Wanner C, Zidek W: Review on uremic toxins: classification, concentration, and interindividual variability. Kidney Int 2003;63:1934–1943.
17 Ward RA: Protein-leaking membranes for hemodialysis: a new class of membranes in search of an application? J Am Soc Nephrol 2005;16:2124–2430.

Ikuto Masakane
Yabuki Shima Clinic
4-5-5 Shima Kita, Yamagata 990-0885 (Japan)
Tel. +81 23 682 8566
E-Mail imasakan.aipod@seieig.or.jp

Saito A, Kawanishi H, Yamashita AC, Mineshima M (eds): High-Performance Membrane Dialyzers.
Contrib Nephrol. Basel, Karger, 2011, vol 173, pp 95–102

Mass Transfer Mechanisms in High-Performance Membrane Dialyzers

Akihiro C. Yamashita

Department of Human and Environmental Science, School of Engineering,
Shonan Institute of Technology, Fujisawa, Kanagawa, Japan

Abstract

Four dialyzers with super-high-flux membrane or high-performance membrane (HPM) with varying packing density of the hollow fiber (*PDF*) from 29.6 to 53.1% were investigated in aqueous in vitro experiments for the purpose of identifying the mass transfer mechanism for three test solutes. Clearances for relatively small test solutes (creatinine and vitamin B_{12}) slowly increased with *PDF* and reached plateau since mass transfer mechanism of these solutes was diffusion limited. However, since unlike classic high-flux dialyzers a considerable amount of internal filtration (>20 ml/min) should occur in super-high-flux dialyzers even under relatively reduced blood and dialysis fluid flow rates, Q_B = 200 ml/min and Q_D = 500 ml/min, it should contribute to enhance the rate of mass transfer especially for those solutes that cannot be easily removed by diffusion, such as β_2-microglobulin or even larger toxic substances. For dialyzers with the HPM a module design becomes even more important for developing novel commercial products.

Cellulosic membranes have been used for removing toxic substances from chronic renal disease patients for the last four decades after switching from cellophane membrane that was sometimes not strong enough for one session of dialysis treatment. On the other hand, synthetic polymeric membrane was first developed in the late 1960s and has become popular these days. The majority of such membranes have a high hydraulic permeability that is usually called 'high flux' in many clinical situations. Since higher hydraulic permeability membranes are known to have higher solute permeability for so-called middle molecules

Table 1. Classification of dialyzers in the Japanese reimbursement system

Class	β_2-MG clearance ml/min	Reimbursement	Membranes
1	<10	low	low-flux
2	≥10 to <30	↓	classic high-flux
3	≥30 to <50	↓	high-flux
4	≥50 to <70	↓	
5	≥70	high	super-high-flux (HPM)

Experimental condtion: $Q_B = 200$ ml/min, $Q_D = 500$ ml/min, $Q_F = 10$ ml/min/m^2.
$A_0 = 1.5$ m^2.
If A_0 is not 1.5 m^2, use of the closest model is recommended. Clearance for β_2-MG [5] under $A_0 = 1.5$ m^2 may be estimated by using the performance evaluation equations with K_oA as a constant.

that have been thought to be more toxic and are more difficult to remove by diffusion [1]. At the same time, many articles have been published concerning the superiority of high-flux membranes from the biocompatibility point of view to classic cellulosic membranes [2]. Then the concept of high-performance membrane (HPM) therefore includes all three characteristics at the same time, i.e. (1) high hydraulic permeability, (2) high solute permeability especially for 'middle molecules', and (3) high biocompatibility.

Currently available commercial dialyzers are classified into five categories in accordance with clearances for β_2-microglobulin (β_2-MG) in the Japanese reimbursement system (table 1). Among them, dialyzers in classes 4 and 5 are the modern HPM or super-high-flux dialyzers, while those in class 1 are the low flux, class 2 are the 'classic' high flux, which is still called 'high flux' worldwide, and class 3 are the 'modern' high-flux dialyzers. More than 90% of Japanese patients are being treated with class 4 or class 5 dialyzers as of the end of 2010. In this article, the difference in mass transfer mechanisms between 'classic' high-flux' dialyzers and the modern HPM or super-high-flux dialyzers are discussed mainly from the engineering point of view.

Materials and Method

Aqueous in vitro dialysis experiments were performed in the following manner [3]. Creatinine (MW 113; Wako Pure Chemical Ind. Co., Osaka, Japan), vitamin B_{12} (MW 1,355; Wako Pure Chemical Ind. Co.), and chymotrypsin (MW 25,000; Sigma-Aldrich,

St. Louis, Mo., USA) were chosen as test solutes. A test solution including one of three test solutes was prepared at 37°C (310 K) with 15 liters of pure water for creatinine and vitamin B_{12}, 2 liters of phosphate buffer solution (pH = 7.4) for chymotrypsin, or with bovine blood, mimicking the clinical situation. Four dialyzers with polyester polymer alloy membrane (numerically calculated membrane surface area A_0 is 1.2 m^2) with varying packing density of the hollow fiber (*PDF*), i.e. 29.6, 35.3, 44.1, and 53.1%, were assembled (by Nikkiso Co., Tokyo, Japan) and were investigated. The test solution (pseudo blood) was pumped from the tank into a dialyzer by a roller pump at a varying flow rate (Q_B = 100, 200, 300, and 400 ml/min) and was returned to the same tank. The dialysis fluid (pure water or phosphate buffer, depending on the solute of interest) flow was operated in the countercurrent manner to the pseudo blood at a varying flow rate (Q_D = 350, 500, and 650 ml/min). The net ultrafiltration rate Q_F was set equal to zero. Aliquot samples were taken at various time intervals from the blood line at the inlet (C_{Bi}) and outlet (C_{Bo}) of the dialyzer as well as from the outlet of the dialysis fluid (C_{Do}). Absorbance of those samples were measured by a spectrophotometer (UV-1600 PC; Shimadzu Co., Kyoto, Japan) for the aqueous system, and by a liquid chromatography (LC-10A; Shimadzu Co.) for the bovine blood system to obtain concentrations.

Theoretical

The definition of *PDF* is the ratio of the cross-sectional area of hollow fibers (based on the outer diameter of the hollow fiber) to that of the superficial cross-sectional area of the dialyzer casing that can be calculated as follows:

$$PDF = \frac{\frac{\pi}{4}(d+2\times\Delta x)^2 \times n}{\frac{\pi}{4}dd^2} = \left(\frac{d+2\times\Delta x}{dd}\right)^2 \times n \tag{1}$$

where d is the inner diameter of the hollow fiber (= 0.021 cm), dd is that of the outer casing (= 3.10, 3.40, 3.80, 4.15 cm), n is the number of hollow fibers (= 7133), and Δx is the thickness of the hollow fiber (= 0.0035 cm). The solute clearance C_L with no net ultrafiltration ($Q_F = 0$) can be defined in the usual manner:

$$C_L = \frac{C_{Bi} - C_{Bo}}{C_{Bi}} \times Q_B \tag{2}$$

Diffusion performance of the mass transfer can be characterized by an engineering parameter, the overall mass transfer-area coefficient, that is a product of the overall mass transfer coefficient K_o and the effective membrane surface area A and can be calculated by the following equation [5]:

$$K_o A = \frac{1}{\frac{1}{Q_B} - \frac{1}{Q_D}} \times \ln\left(\frac{1-\frac{C_L}{Q_D}}{1-\frac{C_L}{Q_B}}\right) \tag{3}$$

The internal filtration [4], the ultrafiltration from blood compartment to dialysis fluid compartment and its reverse filtration from dialysis fluid to blood, was mathematically analyzed by using a set of differential equations shown in the Appendix.

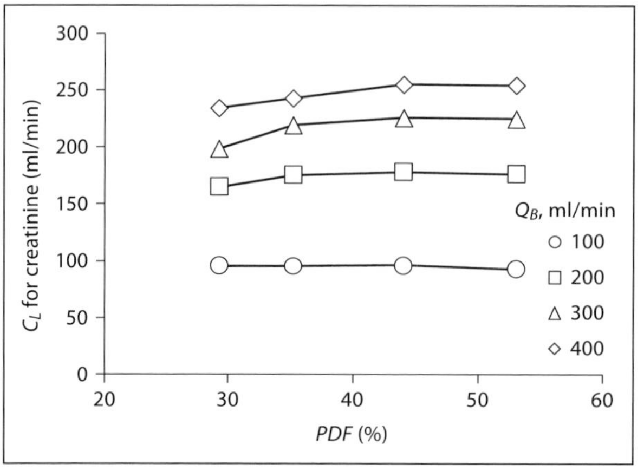

Fig. 1. Relationship between C_L for creatinine and *PDF* (Q_D = 500 ml/min, *n* = 3).

Results and Discussion

Clearances for creatinine under the conditions of Q_D = 500 ml/min and varying Q_B are shown in figure 1. Clearances increased with the increase of *PDF* from 29.6 to 35.3% when $Q_B \geq 200$ ml/min and they increased relatively more gradually in the *PDF* range of 35.3 and 53.1%. Results for vitamin B_{12} were similar to those of creatinine with a little higher increase rate in clearances with the increase of *PDF* (data not shown). Since diffusion is thought to be the dominant mechanism for removing these relatively small solutes, a *PDF* of 29.6% may be too low in terms of removing diffusion dominating solutes due to less likelihood of dialysis fluid contacting the membrane.

On the contrary, C_L for chymotrypsin fairly abruptly increased in a convex fashion rather than reaching a certain value when *PDF* was >44.1% (fig. 2). The K_oA values for chymotrypsin under 12 different flow conditions were then computed and are shown in figure 3 as a function of *PDF*. The K_oA values were almost constant to 55 ml/min on the average in the *PDF* range of 29.6–44.1%, and an even more abrupt increase of K_oA (as high as 120 ml/min when *PDF* was 53.1%) than that in clearance was observed. As one would theoretically and easily imagine, both K_o and A are functions of Q_D and Q_B; therefore, it is natural that the value of K_oA increases with the increase of Q_D and Q_B. However, the abrupt increase of K_oA found with the increase of *PDF* cannot be directly explained by the classic diffusion theory.

A computer simulation was made for analyzing the system with a rigorous mathematical model that includes the effect of internal filtration [4]. Theoretical results in the case of *PDF* = 53.1% with a product of the hydraulic

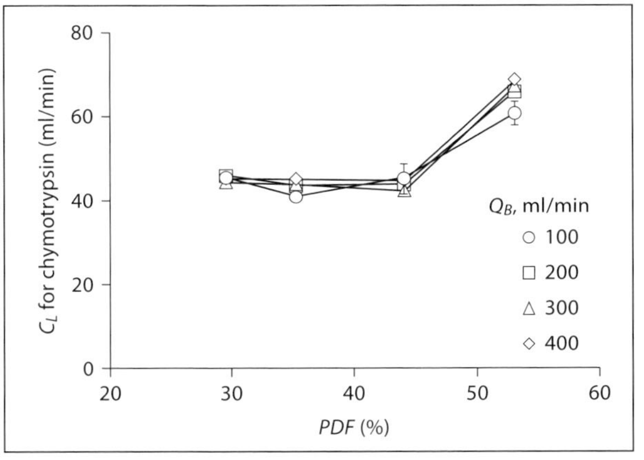

Fig. 2. Relationship between C_L for chymotrypsin and *PDF* (Q_D = 500 ml/min, n = 3).

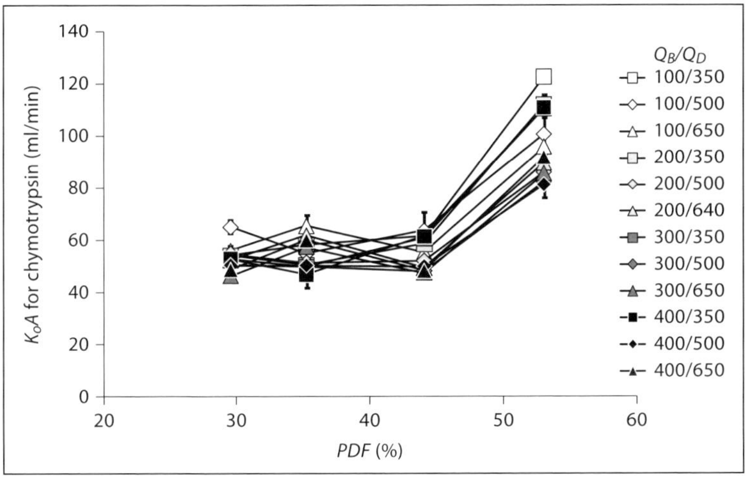

Fig. 3. Relationship between K_OA for chymotrypsin and *PDF*.

permeability Lp and the effective surface area A, LpA = 510 ml/h/mm Hg (super-high-flux) and with LpA = 20.4 ml/h/mm Hg ('classic' high-flux) are shown in figure 4. Both Q_B and Q_D are unchanged throughout the dialyzer in the 'classic' high-flux dialyzer (fig. 4b); however, they are expected to be greatly changed as much as 32 ml/min in the super-high-flux dialyzer (fig. 4a) just by flowing blood and dialysis fluid at rates of 200 and 500 ml/min, respectively. Due to approximately 30 ml/min of bulk flow across the membrane, the

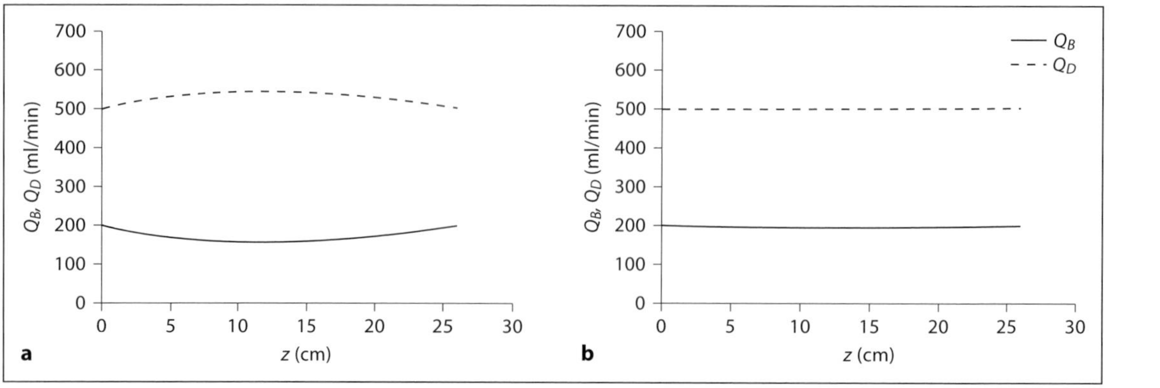

Fig. 4. Computed results of internal filtration distribution in a dialyzer with PDF of 53.1%. **a** Super-high-flux membrane (*LpA* = 360 ml/h/mm Hg). **b** 'Classic' high-flux membrane (*LpA* = 21.6 ml/h/mm Hg).

mass transfer may be increased if the membrane has suitable pores to penetrate across for those solutes that cannot be easily diffused across the membrane. Therefore not only the high hydraulic permeability but also high sieving coefficients for those solutes are important to increase the mass transfer by internal filtration. Under such circumstance, and according to figures 2 and 3, the internal filtration may greatly enhance the mass transfer even beyond the region where the diffusion no longer contributes to mass transfer, which explains the abrupt increase of C_L with the increase of *PDF*. Moreover, what is important is that unlike 'classic' high-flux dialyzers, a considerable amount of internal filtration (>30 ml/min) may be expected in super-high-flux dialyzers even under relatively reduced flow rates, $Q_B = 200$ ml/min and $Q_D = 500$ ml/min, although the effect may be greatly diminishing over time due to the membrane fouling in clinical situations.

Conclusions

Mass transfer across the membrane of relatively small solutes is controlled by diffusion and cannot be influenced much by the performance of the dialyzer. On the contrary, unlike the 'classic' high-flux dialyzers, a considerable amount of internal filtration (>30 ml/min) may be expected in super-high-flux dialyzers even under relatively reduced flow rates, $Q_B = 200$ ml/min and $Q_D = 500$ ml/min. The internal filtration contributes to the enhancement of the rate of mass transfer or increasing clearances for those solutes that cannot be removed by diffusion with ease, such as β_2-MG or even larger toxic substances. For the super-high-flux membranes (HPM), a module design, including the packing density of the hollow fiber, *L/dd* ratio of the module, becomes even more important for the production of commercial dialyzers because the design is directly related to the amount of internal filtration.

Appendix

Considering a realistic situation, a rigorous approach may be necessary and amount of internal filtration may be computed [6] using the following equations:

$$\frac{dP_B(z)}{dz}=-\frac{128\cdot\mu_B(z)}{\pi\cdot d^4\cdot n}\times Q_B(z) \tag{4}$$

$$\frac{dP_D(z)}{dz}=\frac{32\cdot\mu_D}{d_e^{\,2}\cdot S_D}\times Q_D(z) \tag{5}$$

$$\frac{dQ_B(z)}{dz}=-\frac{dQ_D(z)}{dz}=-L_p\cdot\left(\frac{A}{L}\right)\cdot\left\{P_B(z)-P_D(z)-\Delta\pi\right\} \tag{6}$$

$$d_e=\frac{dd^2+(d+2\times\Delta x)^2\times n}{dd+(d+2\times\Delta x)\times n} \tag{7}$$

$$S_D=\frac{\pi}{4}\left\{dd^2-(d+2\times\Delta x)^2\times n\right\} \tag{8}$$

$$\Delta\pi=2.1\times C_p+0.16\times C_p^{\,2}+0.009\times C_p^{\,3} \qquad (9)\ [7]$$

where C_P is the total protein concentration in blood (= 7.0 g/dl) [g/dl], d_e is the equivalent diameter for the dialysis fluid [cm], L is the effective length of the hollow fiber (= 25.5 cm), L_p is the hydraulic permeability of the membrane [cm/min/mmHg], $P_B(z)$ and $P_D(z)$ are pressure distributions in blood and in dialysis fluid in a dialyzer [mmHg], respectively, S_D is the cross-sectional area of dialysis fluid flow [cm^2], $\mu_B(z)$ and μ_D are the viscosities in blood and in dialysis fluid at 310 K [g/cm/s] ($\mu_B(z) = \mu_D$ = constant for aqueous system), respectively, Δx is the thickness of the hollow fiber (= 0.0035 cm), and $\Delta\pi$ is the oncotic pressure due to protein molecules [mmHg]. (Note that an appropriate unit conversion factor is necessary for pressure calculation.) This set of ordinary differential equations can be numerically solved by the fourth-order Runge-Kutta technique to evaluate the rate of internal filtration.

References

1 Babb AL, Popovich RP, Christopher TG, Scribner BH: The genesis of the square meter-hour hypothesis. Trans Am Soc Artif Intern Organs 1971;17:81–91.
2 Hakim RM, Fearon DT, Lazarus J M, Perzanowski CS: Biocompatibility of dialysis membranes: effects of chronic complement activation. Kidney Int 1984;26:194–200.
3 Japanese Society for Artificial Organs: Guideline for Performance Evaluation of Dialyzers (in Japanese). Tokyo, JSAO, 1982.
4 Dellanna F, Wuepper A, Baldamus CA: Internal filtration – advantage in haemodialysis? Nephrol Dial Transplant 1996;11(suppl 2):83–86.
5 Michaels AS: Operating parameters and performance criteria for hemodialyzers and other membrane-separation devices. Trans Am Soc Artif Intern Organs 1966;12:387–392.
6 Yamashita A: New dialysis membrane for removal of middle molecule uremic toxins, Am J Kidney Dis 2001;38(suppl 1):S217–S219.
7 Landis EM, Pappenheimer JR: Handbook of Physiology, Section 2: Circulation. Washington, American Physiological Society, 1986, vol 2, chapt 29.

Akihiro C. Yamashita, PhD
Department of Human and Environmental Science
School of Engineering, Shonan Institute of Technology
1-1-25 Tsujido-Nishikaigan, Fujisawa, Kanagawa 251-8511 (Japan)
Tel./Fax +81 466 300234, E-Mail yama@la.shonan-it.ac.jp

Saito A, Kawanishi H, Yamashita AC, Mineshima M (eds): High-Performance Membrane Dialyzers.
Contrib Nephrol. Basel, Karger, 2011, vol 173, pp 103–109

Fluid and Solute Transfer Characteristics in a Dialyzer with a High-Performance Membrane

Michio Mineshima

Department of Clinical Engineering, Tokyo Women's Medical University, Tokyo, Japan

Abstract

To date, many types of high-flux dialyzers with high-performance membranes have been developed. They seem to have a higher internal filtration flow rate (Q_{IF}) because of a higher ultrafiltration coefficient. In the health reimbursement system in Japan, commercially available dialyzers are categorized into five types based on their β_2-microglobulin clearance (K_{BMG}) values. Although the K_{BMG} value was not correlated strongly with the Q_{IF} value for 26 types of commercially available dialyzers, almost all the dialyzers with a higher Q_{IF} value had a higher K_{BMG} value. These dialyzers seem to have a higher convective transport because of internal filtration in addition to diffusive transport. We measured the blood flow velocity in a cross-sectional plane of the dialyzer using pulse Doppler ultrasonography to evaluate Q_{IF}. It is a useful method for the bedside monitoring because it is noninvasive to the patient and produces reliable data with a higher reproducibility. On the other hand, membrane fouling occurs more easily in higher Q_{IF} dialyzers, compared with conventional dialyzers, because of the higher degree of membrane fouling. Internal filtration-enhanced hemodialysis (IFEHD) using these dialyzers, therefore, has the advantage of increasing solute removal efficiency by enhancing convective transport and the simultaneous disadvantage of decreasing solute removal efficiency by causing membrane fouling. Thus, IFEHD treatment should be performed using a dialyzer with a high-performance membrane to ensure that the advantage is superior to the disadvantage.

The fluid and solute transfer performances of dialyzers have been improved as a result of advances in membrane and device technology. To date, many types of dialyzers with high-performance membranes have been developed.

In some of these dialyzers, the pressure drop in the blood and dialysate streams occurs in a countercurrent manner, inducing internal filtration/backfiltration

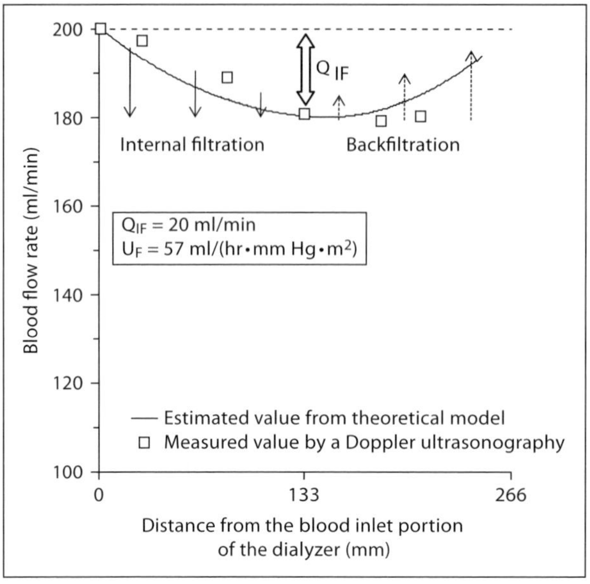

Fig. 1. Q_B profile along a dialyzer and estimation of the Q_{IF}.

(IF/BF) as shown in figure 1. Namely, when the net filtration of the dialyzer is low, filtration from the blood through the membrane and to the dialysate occurs in the upstream of the blood flow and BF from the dialysate to the blood occurs in the downstream. Many types of high-flux dialyzers with high-performance membranes seem to have a high IF/BF flow rate.

In the health reimbursement system in Japan, commercially available dialyzers are categorized into five types based on their β_2-microglobulin clearance (K_{BMG}) values, namely: category I consists of dialyzers with K_{BMG} <10 ml/min, category II consists of dialyzers with $10 \leq K_{BMG} <30$, category III consists of dialyzers with $30 \leq K_{BMG} <50$, category IV consists of dialyzers with $50 \leq K_{BMG} <70$, and category V consists of dialyzers with $70 \leq K_{BMG}$.

Figure 2 shows the relationship between the K_{BMG} value and the internal filtration flow rate (Q_{IF}) defined as the inlet blood flow rate minus the minimum blood flow rate (as shown in figure 1), for 26 types of commercially available dialyzers made in Japan [1]. Although a strong correlation was not obtained, almost all the dialyzers with a higher Q_{IF} value had a higher K_{BMG} value. These dialyzers seem to have a higher convective transport because of IF in addition to diffusive transport.

Effects of Internal Filtration on Dialyzer Performance

In 1996, Dellanna et al. [2] reported the clinical application of dialyzers designed for enhanced IF as a means of increasing solute clearance. The enhanced IF in

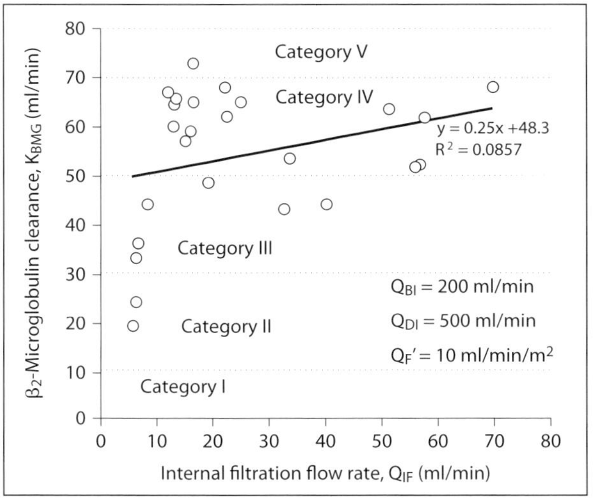

Fig. 2. A relationship between K_{BMG} and Q_{IF} for 26 types of commercially available dialyzers made in Japan [1].

these dialyzers increases the convective transport of the solute in addition to the diffusive transport. We examined the effects of IF on the efficiency of solute removal using analytical and experimental studies [3]. The results of the analytical study showed that although the IF seemed to be affected by several parameters, namely the blood flow rate (Q_B), dialysate flow rate (Q_D), the patient's hematocrit level, the patient's plasma total protein level, and the effective length (L_{eff}), inner diameter (D), and density ratio (DR) of the hollow fibers, the Q_{IF} value increased markedly at a smaller D, a longer L_{eff}, and larger DR values. Meanwhile, an in vitro evaluation using a myoglobin solution showed the same tendencies as in the analytical study.

Internal filtration-enhanced hemodialysis (IFEHD) seems to be more effective and convenient than hemodiafiltration therapy, since IFEHD requires no additional equipment such as a roller pump. However, since the Q_{IF} values of the dialyzers have never been precisely evaluated, no clear estimates of their solute removal characteristics have been made, and selecting the operating conditions for IFEHD treatment has been difficult.

We measured the blood flow velocity in a cross-sectional plane of the dialyzer using pulse Doppler ultrasonography to evaluate the Q_{IF} [4, 5], namely the blood flow velocity through a cross-sectional plane of the dialyzer was directly measured along the dialyzer during a bovine in vitro study using a newly developed probe slider. The plots in figure 1 show the measured values for Q_{IF} using this method.

Since 1992, Ronco's group has performed several studies to estimate IF along dialyzers using a gamma camera [6, 7] and a computerized helical scanning

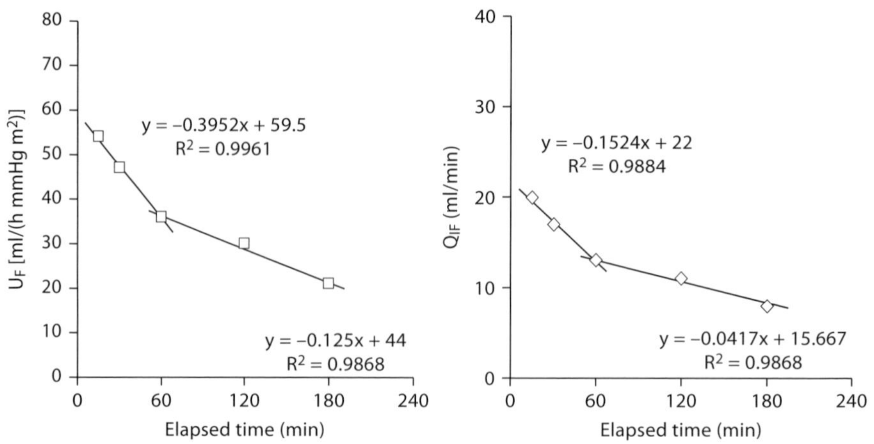

Fig. 3. Time course of U_F and Q_{IF} during a bovine in vitro study.

technique [8, 9], while Hardy et al. [10] measured the local ultrafiltration flow rates in dialyzers using magnetic resonance imaging. Although excellent data were obtained for several dialyzers, these methods are somewhat complicated and cannot be used in clinical practice. The Doppler ultrasonography method that we introduced, on the other hand, is a useful method for the bedside monitoring of the Q_{IF} of dialyzers because it is noninvasive to the patient and produces reliable data with a higher reproducibility. Indeed, we have used this technique in clinical situations.

Time Decay in Dialyzer Performance

As shown in figure 3, the time courses of ultrafiltration coefficient (U_F: ml/(h mmHg m^2)) and the Q_{IF} values were examined during a bovine in vitro study. These values decreased with time after the start of the experiment. These tendencies to decrease, however, exhibit two phases: a relatively rapid drop within 60 min, and a slow decrease thereafter. Thus, two processes that foul the dialyzer seem to occur during hemodialysis treatment. Furthermore, the α_1-microglobulin clearance (K) value gradually decreased and the albumin K value steeply decreased with time, although the creatinine and β_2-microglobulin K values remained nearly constant over time during the course of the experiment, as shown in figure 4 [11]. The result was likely observed because α_1-microglobulin transfer through the membrane is strongly affected by membrane fouling.

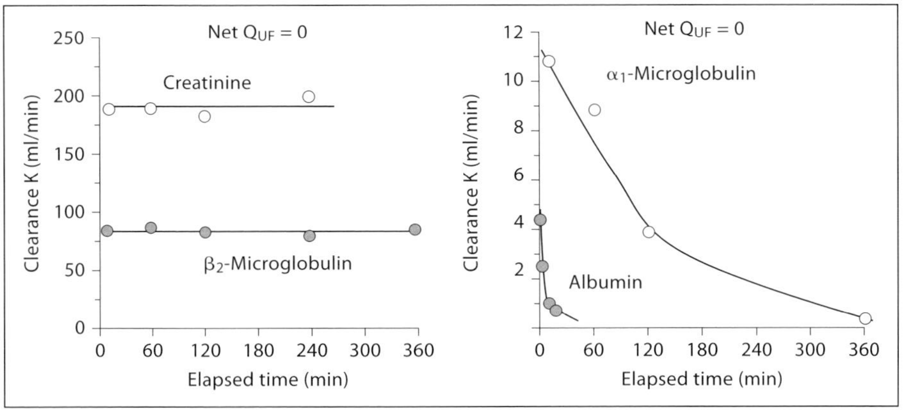

Fig. 4. Time courses of creatinine and β_2-microglobulin, α_1-microglobulin and albumin clearances during a bovine in vitro study [11]. Dialyzer: APS-15E (Asahi Kasei Kuraray Medical Co. Ltd; Polysulfone, A = 1.5 m^2).

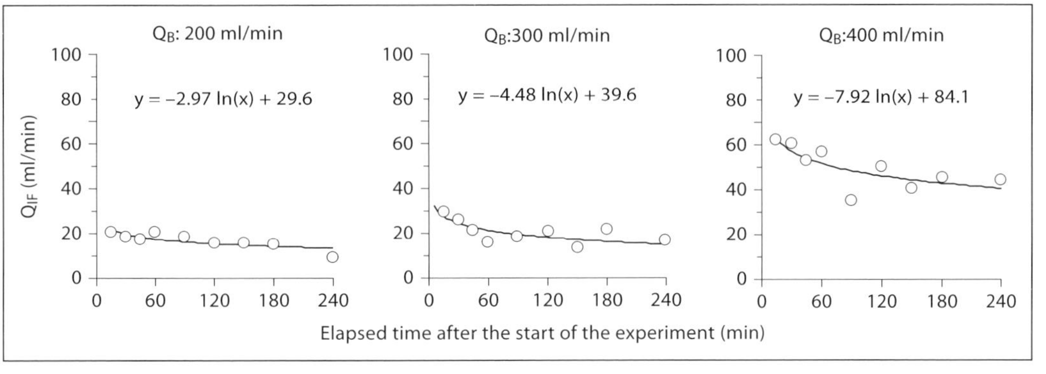

Fig. 5. Time courses of the Q_{IF} at different Q_B for APS-15SA. Dialyzer: APS-15SA (Asahi Kasei Kuraray Medical Co. Ltd; Polysulfone, A = 1.5 m^2).

Effect of Blood Flow Rate on Internal Filtration

Figure 5 shows the time courses of the Q_{IF} values at different Q_B for APS-15SA (Asahi Kasei Kuraray Medical Co. Ltd; Polysulfone, A = 1.5 m^2), which is a category IV dialyzer. These results were obtained using ultrasonography in a bovine in vitro study. Table 1 shows the total IF over 4 h estimated using the time course of the measured Q_{IF} values. At a higher Q_B, a higher time-averaged Q_{IF} value was obtained, but the Q_{IF} value decreased more with time because of the higher degree of membrane fouling.

Table 1. Total IF (liters) over 4 h

Q_B, ml/min	Total V_{IF}, l
200	3.77
300	4.50
400	11.3

Dialyzer: APS-15SA (Asahi Kasei Kuraray Medical Co. Ltd, Polysulfone, A = 1.5 m^2).

In an enhanced IF dialyzer, the pressure drop on the blood side is relatively higher than that in conventional dialyzers. Membrane fouling occurs more easily in enhanced IF dialyzers, compared with conventional dialyzers, because the local transmembrane pressure adjacent to the inlet of the blood flow is relatively high to enhance the IF. IFEHD, therefore, has the advantage of increasing solute removal efficiency by enhancing convective transport and the simultaneous disadvantage of decreasing solute removal efficiency by causing membrane fouling. Thus, IFEHD treatment should be performed using a dialyzer with a high-performance membrane to ensure that the advantage is superior to the disadvantage.

Conclusions

Many types of high-flux dialyzers with high-performance membranes seem to have a higher Q_{IF} because of a higher U_F. These dialyzers have higher solute transfer characteristics based on the convective transport caused by IF in addition to the diffusive transport. However, membrane fouling occurs more easily in these dialyzers than in conventional dialyzers. Consequently, adequate operation of a dialyzer with a high-performance membrane is required for effective usage in individual patients.

References

1 Akiba T, Kawanishi H, Mineshima M, et al: Guidelines for dialysate quality and performance evaluation of blood purification devices in 2008 (in Japanese). J Jpn Soc Dial Ther 2008;41:159–167.

2 Dellanna F, Wuepper A, Baldamus CA: Internal filtration – advantage in haemodialysis? Nephrol Dial Transplant 1996;11 (suppl 2):83–86.

3 Mineshima M, Ishimori I, Ishida K, Hoshino T, Kaneko I, Sato Y, Agishi T, Tamamura N, Sakurai H, Masuda T, Hattori H: Effects of internal filtration on the solute removal efficiency of a dialyzer. ASAIO J 2000;46: 456–460.
4 Sato Y, Mineshima M, Ishimori I: Effect of hollow fiber length on solute removal and quantification of internal filtration rate by Doppler ultrasound. Int J Artif Organs 2003; 26:129–134.
5 Mineshima M: Estimation of internal filtration flow rate in high-flux dialyzers by Doppler ultrasonography. Hemodiafiltation – a new era. Contrib Nephrol. Basel, Karger, 2011, vol 168, pp 153–161.
6 Ronco C, Brendolan A, Feriani M, Milan M, Conz P, Lupi A, Berto P, Bettini M, La Greca G: A new scintigraphic method to characterize ultrafiltration in hollow fiber dialyzers. Kidney Intl 1992;41:1383–1393.
7 Ronco C, Brendolan A, Lupi A, Metry G, Levin NW: Effects of a reduced inner diameter of hollow fibers in hemodialyzers. Kidney Int 2000;58:809–817.
8 Ronco C, Brendolan A, Crepaldi C, Rodighiero M, Everard P, Ballestri M, Cappelli G, Spittle M, La Greca G: Dialysate flow distribution in hollow fiber hemodialyzers with different dialysate pathway configurations. Int J Artif Organs 2000;23:601–609.
9 Ronco C, Brendolan A, Crepaldi C, Rodighiero M, Scabardi M: Blood and dialysate flow distributions in hollow-fiber hemodialyzers analyzed by computerized helical scanning technique. J Am Soc Nephrol 2002;13(suppl 1):S53–S61.
10 Hardy PA, Poh CK, Liao Z, Clark WR, Gao D: The use of magnetic resonance imaging to measure the local ultrafiltration rate in hemodialyzers. J Membr Sci 2002;204: 195–205.
11 Mineshima M, Ishimori I, Sakiyama R: Validity of internal filtration-enhanced hemodialysis as a new hemodiafiltration therapy. Blood Purif 2009;27:33–37.

Dr. Michio Mineshima
Department of Clinical Engineering, Tokyo Women's Medical University
8-1, Kawada-cho, Shinjuku-ku, Tokyo 162-8666 (Japan)
Tel. +81 3 3353 8112, ext. 37203
E-Mail mmine@ce.twmu.ac.jp

Saito A, Kawanishi H, Yamashita AC, Mineshima M (eds): High-Performance Membrane Dialyzers.
Contrib Nephrol. Basel, Karger, 2011, vol 173, pp 110–118

Contribution of Polysulfone Membranes to the Success of Convective Dialysis Therapies

Sudhir K. Bowry · Emanuele Gatti · Jörg Vienken

BioSciences, Fresenius Medical Care Deutschland GmbH, Bad Homburg, Germany

Abstract

The majority of patients with chronic kidney disease are currently treated with dialyzers containing synthetic membranes. Of all the dialysis membranes made from these polymers, 93% are from the parent polyarylsulfone family of which 71% are from polysulfone (PSu) and 22% from polyethersulfone. The preference of nephrologists for PSu dialyzers signifies their versatility in terms of meeting the solute and fluid removal demands for all treatment modalities (low- and high-flux dialysis, online hemodiafiltration, hemofiltration). The unprecedented success and widespread usage of PSu membranes is attributed, in addition to efficient removal of a broad spectrum of uremic toxins, to other criteria required of modern dialysis therapies. Namely, effective endotoxin retention capacity, pronounced intrinsic biocompatibility and low cytotoxicity are factors which all contribute to minimal adverse clinical sequelae. Furthermore, PSu by virtue of its high thermal stability can be sterilized with steam, the preferred mode of sterilization as it does not have the disadvantages associated with other sterilization methods. However, there are significant differences between membranes made from PSu due to differences in membrane polymer recipes and manufacturing technologies. Although PSu may be the main constituent, these membranes are blended with other polymers, e.g. hydrophilizing agents, such as polyvinylpyrrolidone to give each membrane its characteristic profile. The relative amounts of the two (or more) co-polymers as well as the spinning conditions provide a fingerprint of each membrane in terms of solute separation characteristics, biocompatibility, cytotoxicity or endotoxin retention capabilities. PSu membrane-based dialyzers thus fulfill the crucial therapy requirements of current treatment modalities to varying extents. Thereby, different effects towards patient outcomes and treatment safety are achieved.

The selection of the polymer material for the fabrication of dialysis membranes has significant implications on the quality of hemodialysis (HD) therapy delivered to patients with chronic kidney disease (CKD) [1]. Only a limited number of polymer materials are suitable for the spinning and extrusion processes involved in the manufacture of hollow-fiber membranes. The selection of polymers was originally based on experiences from textile fiber production. Clinical experience has shown that modern dialysis membranes need to meet certain key requirements, thereby further limiting the number of polymers for contemporary dialysis therapies [2]. Throughout the progression of HD as a routine therapy, membrane polymer types have evolved essentially in line with clinical observations and constantly changing clinical requirements.

Polysulfone (PSu) belongs to a family of thermoplastic polymers which are known for their chemical and thermal stability. They contain the subunits 'aryl-SO_2-aryl' and 'benzyl-SO_2-benzyl' (fig. 1), of which the sulfone (SO_2) group provides the name for the polymer. Ever since the first PSu-based membrane became available for routine dialysis in 1984, there has been a steady increase in the application of PSu membranes in dialysis [3]. 93% of all dialysis membranes in current use are from the parent polyarylsulfone family of which 71% are from PSu and 22% from polyethersulfone (Fresenius Medical Care Market Analysis 2010, unpubl. data). The unprecedented success and widespread usage of PSu-based dialyzers is attributed to appropriate and efficient solute and fluid removal capabilities as well as an effective endotoxin retention capacity. Moreover, a pronounced intrinsic biocompatibility combined with a low cytotoxicity leads to low levels of adverse clinical sequelae that can be further alleviated by the preferred steam sterilization mode. The PSu polymer fulfils a decisive need for medical devices, i.e. high thermal stability with a glass transition temperature of T_G >190°C. PSu lends itself to sterilization by steam. PSu is also highly stable towards most chemical agents. It is important to note that there are significant differences between membranes made from PSu due to differences in membrane manufacturing technology – analogous to the creation of highly individual culinary fares from the same combination of ingredients but according to unique recipes.

Factors Contributing to the Acceptance of PSu Dialysis Membranes

In 1985, shortly after PSu dialyzers became available for routine clinical application, over 85% of all dialysis treatments were carried out with cellulose membrane-based dialyzers [4]. Today, a quarter of a century later, a complete reversal has taken place with under 15% of dialysis being conducted with cellulosic dialyzers. The major producer of cellulose dialyzer membranes (Membrana GmbH, Wuppertal, Germany, the manufacturer of Cuprophan® and Hemophan®) even ceased its production in 2006. This dramatic shift of perceptions can be

The PSu material

Raw material:	Udel P-1,700 (Solvay)
Maximum temperature:	175–180°C
Glass transition temperature:	190°C
Density:	1.24 g/cm^3

Polysulfone

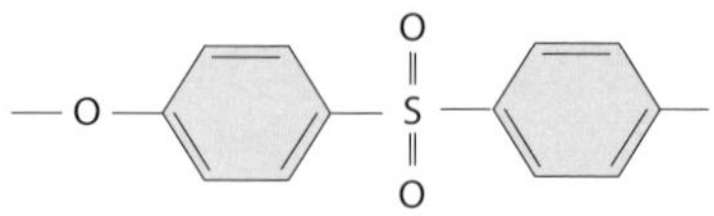

Polyethersulfone (PES)
(Poly-aryl-ethersulfone (PAES)

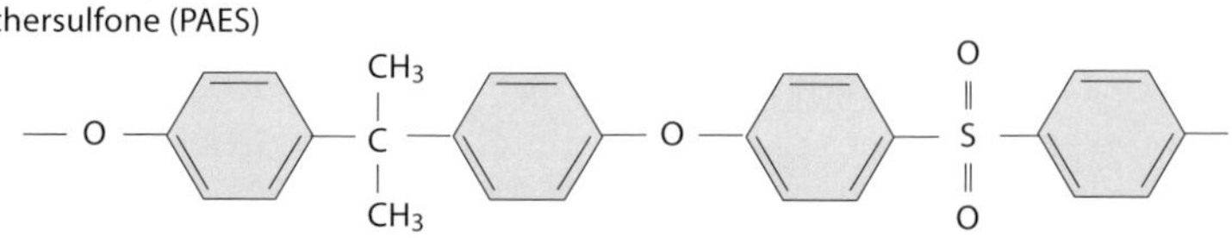

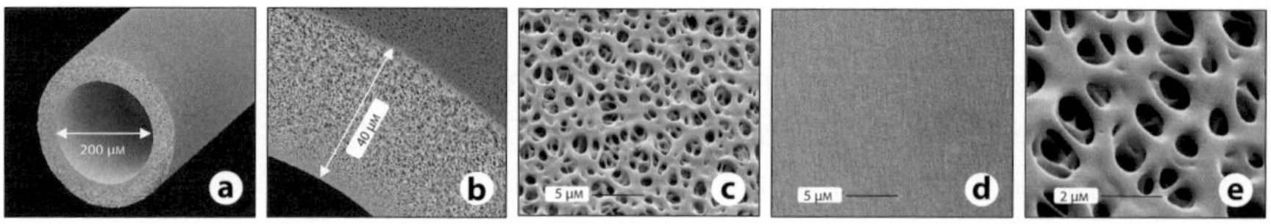

Fig. 1. Chemical structure and characteristics of PSu polymers used for dialysis membranes. The chemical structure is based on the 'benzyl-SO_2-benzyl' group. Benzene rings are considered to interact with LPS molecules and facilitate their adsorption. Not all PSu membranes are alike as an aryl-SO_2-aryl group may be added to the sulfone molecule and thus form polyarylethersulfones (PAES). The lower panel shows (**a**) a cross section of a PSu capillary membrane (internal diameter, x: 185–200 µm), (**b**) a cross section of the membrane wall (overall wall thickness, y: 35–40 µm), (**c**) view of the inner membrane surface (bar: 5 µm), and (**d**) view of the outer membrane surface (bar: 5 µm), and (**e**) view on the outer membrane surface (enlarged, bar: 2 µm). The capillary membrane is composed of a inner 'skin' region of under 1 µm in thickness, the remainder being the support structure needed to maintain its mechanical stability.

attributed essentially to the combination of a better understanding of uremic toxicity and the need to improve dialysis patient survival rates which still remain poor. While dialysis membranes from other polymers may adequately meet the desired individual criteria, most PSu dialysis membranes are able to fulfill the following requirements which, collectively, conform to contemporary therapy practices and needs.

Biocompatibility
From a historical perspective, the initial criterion for the success of PSu membranes can be ascribed to the higher degree of biocompatibility offered by PSu compared to cellulose-based membranes. Membranes made from 'pure' cellulose

caused leukopenia and complement activation which led to the biocompatibility controversy and debate and the demand for better membranes which did not activate these biological pathways [5]. Despite the subsequent development of substituted (or modified) cellulosic membranes with a significant improvement of biocompatibility parameters, the biocompatibility standards already set by PSu membranes could not be surpassed [2, 4].

Elimination of a Broad Spectrum of Uremic Toxins
Removal of retained water and accumulated uremic retention solutes from the blood of uremic patients remains the fundamental feature of all dialysis treatment modalities. While there is the implication of uremic retention solutes with larger molecular weight ('middle molecule' hypothesis), subsequent scientific research on uremic toxicity has established the imperative of removing substances approaching the size of albumin [6]. These larger uremic toxins, together with some smaller uremic toxins that are bound to proteins, need to be removed by high-flux membranes, that is, membranes having higher sieving coefficients for specified substances. PSu is ideally suited for the manufacture of membranes with variable and larger pore sizes, thereby facilitating the efficient removal of large uremic retention solutes that contribute to the uremic syndrome.

Transport
The versatility of PSu as a dialysis membrane material can be attributed to the fact that membrane structures can be tailored to desired specifications. In addition to the higher sieving, increased hydraulic permeability enables efficient transport mechanisms through solvent drag (convection). High ultrafiltration is required for advanced treatment modalities such as online hemodiafiltration (OL-HDF). Solvent drag through high ultrafiltration is the main driving force of OL-HDF therapy in which large quantities of fluid are removed from the patient across high-flux membranes [7]. The overall effect is a more efficient removal of larger uremic toxins as compared to low-flux treatment modes which relies more on diffusion (rather than convection) for solute removal (fig. 2). There is evidence indicating that patients treated with high-flux dialysis and OL-HDF therapy have better survival rates and show fewer complications [8, 9].

Endotoxin Adsorptive Capacity
Dialysis therapies, particularly high-volume OL-HDF, expose the patients to large volumes of substitution fluids. Should these fluids be contaminated with endotoxins (chemically lipopolysaccharides, LPS, derived from the outer wall of Gram-negative bacteria during cell growth and lysis), there is a risk of these substances entering the patient's bloodstream [10]. Endotoxins activate a number of biological pathways, triggering the generation of potent pro-inflammatory substances like cytokines and growth factors [11]. Inflammation,

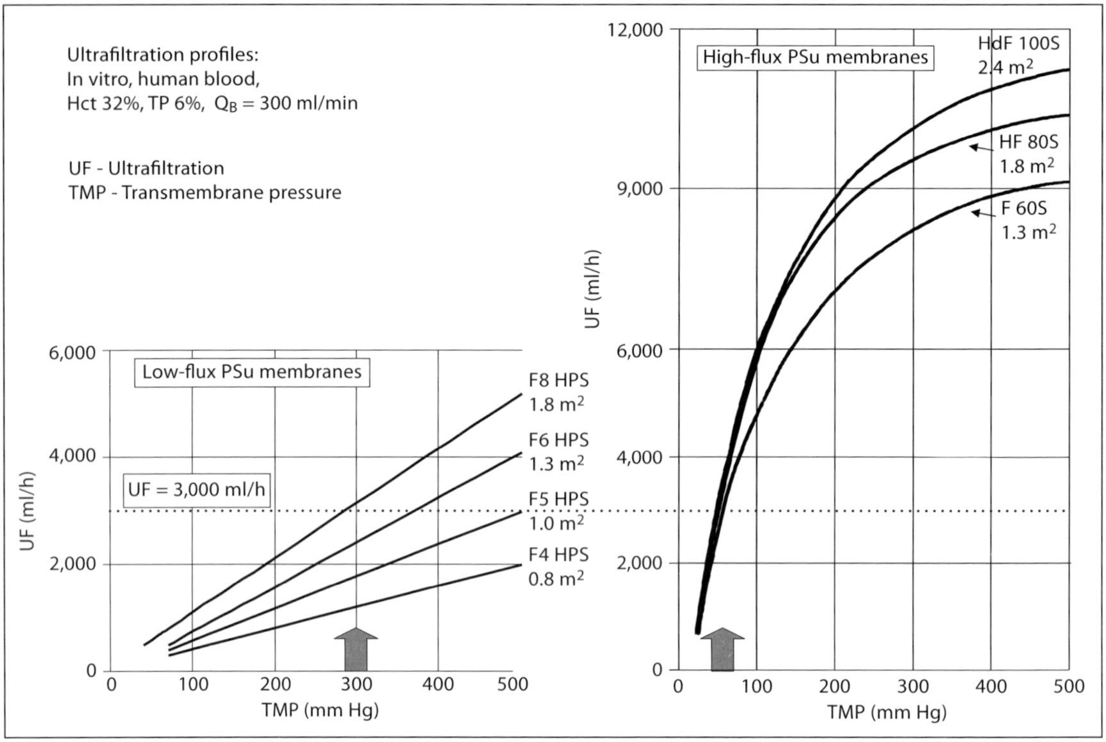

Fig. 2. Ultrafiltration rates (UF/h) with low- and high-flux dialyzers containing PSu membranes. Membrane notations exemplary refer to Fresenius Medical Care's dialyzers (F-series) with different surface areas. Note that a transmembrane pressure (TMP) of 300 mm Hg is needed to achieve an UF rate of 3,000 ml/h with F8HPS (low-flux membrane) and only about 50 mm Hg TMP to obtain the same UF with high-flux membranes.

an underlying mechanism in most diseased states including CKD, is widely recognized to be a major risk factor for cardiovascular disease-related mortality in CKD patients.

Depending on their chemical constitution and microstructure, PSu membranes are able to prevent entry of endotoxins into the patient's blood [12, 13]. Figure 3 shows the endotoxin retention capabilities of diverse PSu dialyzers, each of which was exposed in vitro to the same (high) endotoxin insult in the dialysate compartment [14]. The data demonstrate the fact that dialysis membranes made from different polymers afford highly variable degrees of safety in terms of eliminating endotoxins and curtailing inflammation. Endotoxin adsorption is attributed to a hydrophobic-hydrophobic interaction between the bulk PSu polymer and the endotoxin molecule, that is, the hydrophobic part of the LPS molecule interacts with the hydrophobic part of the PSu structure [11].

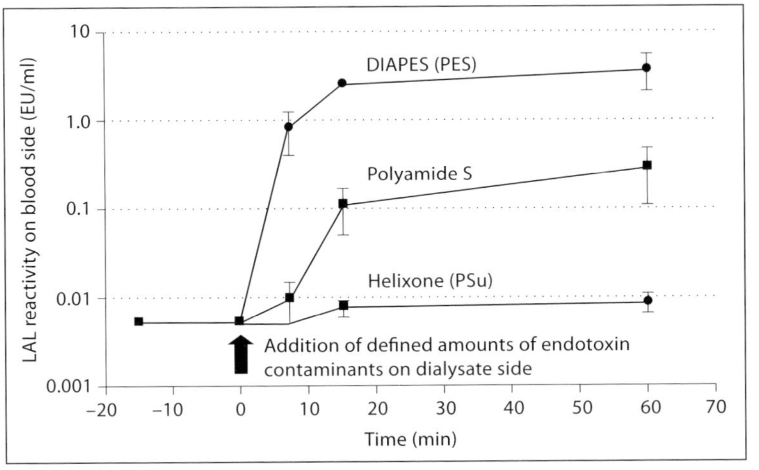

Fig. 3. PSu membranes offer different degrees of safety during dialysis by adsorbing endotoxins from potentially contaminated dialysis fluids. Hydrophobic parts of the lipopolysaccharide (LPS; endotoxin) molecules are considered to interact with hydrophobic entities within the polysulfone structure thereby facilitating their removal. Dialysis membranes have highly variable endotoxin retention capabilities; endotoxin retention to dialysis membranes depends not only on the polymer composition and chemistry but also on the hollow-fibre manufacturing processes. The figure shows the endotoxin activity, as assessed by the *Limulus* amoebocyte lysate (LAL) assay, in the blood compartment of various dialysers after the dialysate compartments were exposed to fluid having the same level of endotoxin contamination.

Key Features and Differences of PSu Membranes

Polymer Composition and Membrane Spinning

When addressing the topic of 'polysulfone' membranes, it is important to recognize that although PSu is the major constituent, these membranes are blends incorporating other polymer materials to give each membrane its characteristic profile. The first PSu-based filters (high-flux, for hemofiltration), was produced solely from a single PSu polymer (example: PSu for hemofilters from the manufacturer Amicon Plastics/USA). PSu itself is hydrophobic, and for its use as an ultrafilter in dialysis it has to be rendered partially hydrophilic, otherwise high transmembrane pressures (TMPs) would be necessary to achieve an adequate ultrafiltration rate (UFR). This is feasible by means of blending the PSu bulk with hydrophilizing agents such as polyvinylpyrrolidone (PVP) or polyethyleneglycol (PEG). Further, and as is now known, the optimal biocompatibility profile of any dialysis membrane is only achieved by the delicate balance of hydrophobic-hydrophilic domains at the blood-contacting surface of the finished product [15]. Thus, membranes made from the polyarylsulfone polymer family (fig. 1), once blended with hydrophilizing co-polymers in an optimal ratio, achieve their final biocompatibility profile already during the production processes. It must be stressed that PVP has an additional role in that it enables the membranes to derive their characteristic structures (in terms of sieving and ultrafiltration properties) during the membrane-spinning process. Depending upon the relative amounts of the two (or more) co-polymers as well as the spinning conditions (e.g. temperature, humidity, time and composition of the coagulation bath), each membrane acquires its own fingerprint in terms of solute separation characteristics, biocompatibility, cytotoxicity or endotoxin retention capabilities [12–14].

Sterilization

Another major reason for the suitability of polyarylsulfone polymers for dialysis membranes is that they can be sterilized with each of the three main sterilization modes used in the medical devices industry: steam, γ-rays and ethylene oxide (ETO) [16]. However, it must be recognized that unlike steam sterilization, both γ-ray and ETO sterilization have been associated with reactions that either may modify the dialyzer materials. A high-energy input following irradiation may destroy or degrade the polymer chain and give rise to extractable oligomers. This alteration of PSu dialyzers by γ-rays may lead to enhanced cytotoxicity (fig. 4) and anaphylactic reactions with ETO-sterilized dialyzers have been observed and documented [17–19].

The high thermal stability of PSu and polyarylsulfones is ideally suited for high-temperature heat or steam sterilization. However, differences in the way steam sterilization is conducted could have significant implications in the effectiveness and hence safety of dialyzers in clinical application. Sterilization of the entire dialyzer with steam may destroy microorganisms but not necessarily eliminate their biologically active components (e.g. LPS). Inline steam sterilization procedures, in which the inner and outer regions of each individual fiber within the dialyzers are flushed with steam at 121°C, ensure that biological material is inactivated and subsequently washed away.

Conclusions

To date, the majority of all the dialysis membranes used worldwide are made from PSu. The prevalence of these dialysis membranes signifies the versatility of PSu in terms of meeting all the performance requirements, particularly in terms of solute and fluid removal for all treatment modalities. Furthermore, as over half of all dialysis treatments worldwide are now carried out with high-flux membranes, PSu membranes, by virtue of their endotoxin retention capabilities, offer a high degree of safety to the patient. PSu dialyzers contribute favorably towards patient outcomes by meeting key aspects of modern dialysis therapies.

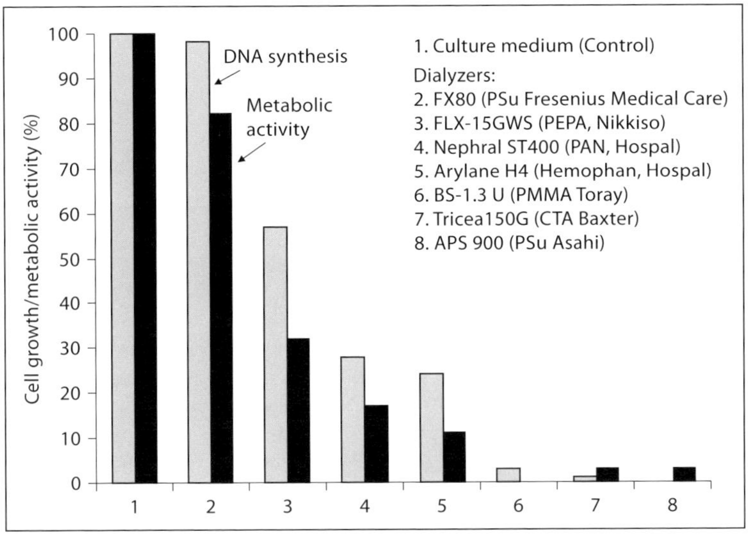

Fig. 4. Comparison of in vitro cytotoxicity evaluation of culture medium as a control (1) and extracts derived from an inline steam sterilized dialyzer (2) and different γ-sterilized dialyzers (3–8). Extracts were derived by incubating the dialyzers with culture medium and thereafter exposed to L929 mouse fibroblast cells. Metabolic activity was measured in triplicate using the tetrazolium salt (WST-1 test reagent) and cell proliferation (as DNA synthesis using the base analogue 5-bromo-2′-deoxyuridine of the BrdU test (colorimetric cell proliferation ELISA BrdU). Reagents for both assays were from Roche Diagnostics, Mannheim, Germany. The readings of the controls (cells incubated with culture medium alone and defined as 100%) were subtracted from those obtained for each extract. PSu = Polysulfone; PEPA = polyester-polymer alloy; PAN = polyacrylonitrile; Hemophan = modified cellulose; PMMA = polymethylmethacrylate; CTA = cellulose triacetate.

References

1 Davenport A: Can dialyzer membrane selection affect outcomes in patients with acute kidney injury requiring dialysis? Hemodial Int 2009;13(suppl 1):S13–S17.

2 Bowry SK: Dialysis membranes today. Intern J Artif Organs 2002;25:447–460.

3 Streicher E, Schneider H: The development of a polysulfone membrane. A new perspective in dialysis? Contrib Nephrol. Basel, Karger, 1985, vol 46, pp 1–13.

4 Vienken J, Diamantoglou M, Henne W, Nederlof B: Artificial dialysis membranes: from concept to large scale production. Am J Nephrol 1999;19:355–362.

5 Kerr PG, Huang L: Membranes for haemodialysis. Nephrology 2010;15:381–385.

6 Glorieux G, Vanholder R: New uremic toxins – which solutes should be removed? Contrib Nephrol. Basel, Karger, 2011, vol 168, pp 117–128.

7 Ledebo I: Convective dialysis therapies, current status and perspective. Ther Apher Dial 2005;9:223–227.

8 Locatelli F, Martin-Malo A, Hannedouche T, Loureiro A, Papadimitriou M, Wizemann V, Jacobson SH, Czekalski S, Ronco C, Vanholder R, Membrane Permeability Outcome (MPO) Study Group: Effect of membrane permeability on survival of hemodialysis patients. J Am Soc Nephrol 2009;20:645–654.

9 Canaud B, Bragg-Gresham JL, Marshall MR, Desmeules S, Gillespie BW, Depner T, Klassen P, Port FK: Mortality risk for patients receiving hemodiafiltration versus hemodialysis: European results from the DOPPS. Kidney Int 2006;69:2087–2093.
10 Schindler R: Inflammation and dialysate quality. Hemodial Int 2006;10:S56–S59.
11 Lonnemann G: Chronic inflammation in hemodialysis: the role of contaminated dialysate. Blood Purif 2000;18:214–23.
12 Henrie M, Ford C, Andersen M, Stroup E, Diaz-Buxo J, Madsen B, Britt D, Ho C: In vitro assessment of dialysis membrane as an endotoxin transfer barrier: geometry, morphology and permeability. Artif Organs 2008;32:701–710.
13 Hayama M, Miyasaki T, Mochizuki S, Asahara H, Tsujioka K, Kohori F, Sakai K, Jinbo Y, Yoshida M: Visualisation of distribution of endotoxin trapped and an endotoxin-blocking filtration membrane. J Membr Sci 2002;210:45–53.
14 Weber V, Linsberger I, Rossmanith E, Weber C, Falkenhagen D: Pyrogen transfer across high- and low-flux hemodialysis membranes. Artif Organs 2004;28:210–217.
15 Vienken J, Diamantoglou M, Hahn C, Kamusewitz H, Paul D: Considerations on developmental aspects of biocompatible dialysis membranes. Artif Organs 1995;19: 398–406.
16 Vienken J: Polymers in nephrology. Characteristics and needs. Int J Artif Organs 2002;25:470–479.
17 Bommer J, Miltenburger H, Hoerner V, Kilian S: Cytotoxicity of γ-ray sterilized dialysis devices (abstract). J Am Soc Nephrol 1994;5:408.
18 Takesawa S, Satoh S, Hidai H, Seikiguchi M, Sakai K: Degradation by γ-irradiation of regenerated cellulose membranes for clinical dialysis. Trans ASAIO 1987;33:584–587
19 Grammer L, Patterson R: IgE against ethylene oxide altered human serum albumin as an etiologic agent in allergic reactions of hemodialysis patients. Artif Organs 1987;11: 97–99.

Dr. Sudhir K. Bowry
Else-Kroenerstrasse 1
BioSciences, Fresenius Medical Care Deutschland GmbH
DE–61352 Bad Homburg (Germany)
Tel. +49 6172 609 2128, E-Mail sudhir.bowry@fmc-ag.com

Mass Transfer Mechanisms and Characteristics of High-Performance Membranes

Saito A, Kawanishi H, Yamashita AC, Mineshima M (eds): High-Performance Membrane Dialyzers.
Contrib Nephrol. Basel, Karger, 2011, vol 173, pp 119–129

AN69: Evolution of the World's First High Permeability Membrane

Michel Thomas[a] · Kazuhiro Moriyama[b] · Ingrid Ledebo[c]

[a]Hospal, Meyzieu, France; [b]Gambro, Tokyo, Japan, and [c]Gambro R&D, Lund, Sweden

Abstract

In response to a request from the French government, Rhône-Poulenc started development of a synthetic membrane for dialysis in 1969. When used for patients the new membrane, AN69, showed improved efficiency and clinical outcome. Treatment times could be reduced, peripheral neuropathy improved and patients expressed improved quality of life. This was the introduction of high-flux, volume-controlled dialysis. The polymer used for the AN69 membrane is a copolymer of acrylonitrile and sodium methallylsulfonate, specially selected for the dialysis application. Contrary to most synthetic membranes AN69 is hydrophilic, because the numerous sulfonate groups attract water and create a hydrogel structure which provides high diffusive and hydraulic permeability. In the AN69 membrane the microstructure and the chemical composition offer a unique context for bulk adsorption of low-molecular-weight proteins, the high water content of the hydrogel making the polymer chains easily accessible. The highly specific adsorptive properties – limited on the surface and favored in the membrane structure and with high specificity for basic, medium-sized proteins – distinguish AN69 from other synthetic high-flux membranes as well as from other so-called adsorptive membranes in the field of dialysis. Since its creation in the early 1970s the AN69 membrane has evolved to meet the requirements and challenges of dialysis therapy. Still the basic characteristics of high permeability to fluid and to a wide range of relevant uremic retention products combined with excellent biocompatibility, whether measured by traditional or novel indicators, have remained the hallmark of the membrane. The unique adsorptive capacity has provided a base for further development. The latest version of AN69, HeprAN, has heparin grafting on the inner surface and enhanced adsorption of bacterial products on the outer surface. Modern versions of AN69 are today used in hemodialysis and contemporary modes of convective therapies for a large number of chronic as well as acute renal patients around the world.

The First Synthetic, High-Flux Membrane

When dialysis developed into a chronic therapy in the 1960s the only membranes available were made of regenerated cellulose. The life-saving impact of the treatment was so overwhelming that the poor efficiency and biocompatibility of the membrane was not an issue.

In 1969, Rhône-Poulenc, a French chemical and pharmaceutical company making membranes for the textile industry, in response to a request from the French government started development of a synthetic membrane for dialysis. In 1972, the first device equipped with the membrane was introduced for clinical use in the Necker Hospital in Paris. This novel membrane was highly permeable not only to large solutes but also to fluid and to permit safe use a new generation of dialysis machines offering accurate volumetric control of ultrafiltration were developed by Rhône-Poulenc. Early reports from studies of dialysis patients treated with the new membrane show improved efficiency and clinical outcome [1]. Treatment times could be reduced, peripheral neuropathy improved and patients expressed improved quality of life. This was the introduction of high-flux, volume-controlled dialysis.

In the early 1970s the Scribner group [2] in Seattle launched the middle molecule hypothesis which emphasized removal of uremic toxins in the range of 500–5,000 Da, so-called middle molecules. The emergence of this concept called for development of dialysis membranes with extended permeability to remove such solutes. It paved the way for the success of the AN69 membrane because all other membranes used at the time were cellulosic and were permeable mainly to small solutes with focus on urea and creatinine. With reference to the birth year and the material, acrylonitrile, the world's first highly permeable dialysis membrane was named AN69. It is important to distinguish the AN69 from other membranes also containing polyacrylonitrile (PAN). The polymer mix in these membranes and thus the character may be quite different and they should not be referred to collectively as PAN membranes. Numerous publications reported significant clinical benefits for patients treated with AN69 filters. The membrane was regarded as 'best in class' and became widely used, especially in southern Europe, Canada and Japan [3].

A Dedicated Polymer and Manufacturing Process

The synthetic polymer used for the AN69 membrane is a copolymer of acrylonitrile and sodium methallylsulfonate, specially selected for the dialysis application (fig. 1). For optimal performance a hemodialysis membrane should have hydrophilic characteristics. Many synthetic polymers used for dialysis membranes are hydrophobic and need to be rendered hydrophilic by addition of water-soluble polymers, e.g. polyvinylpyrrolidone. AN69, however, is

Fig. 1. Chemical formula for AN69 copolymer, consisting of acrylonitrile and sodium methallylsulfonate.

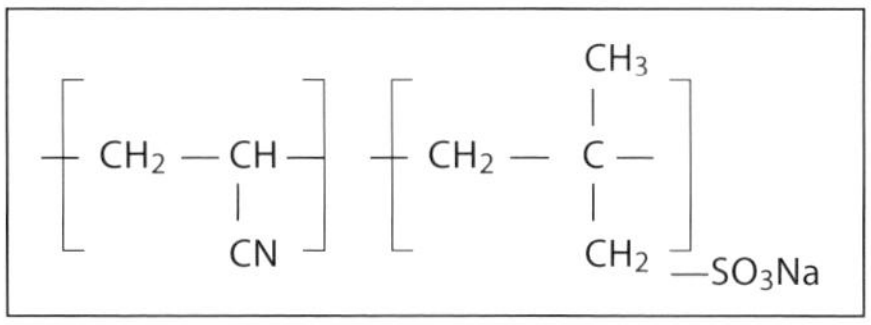

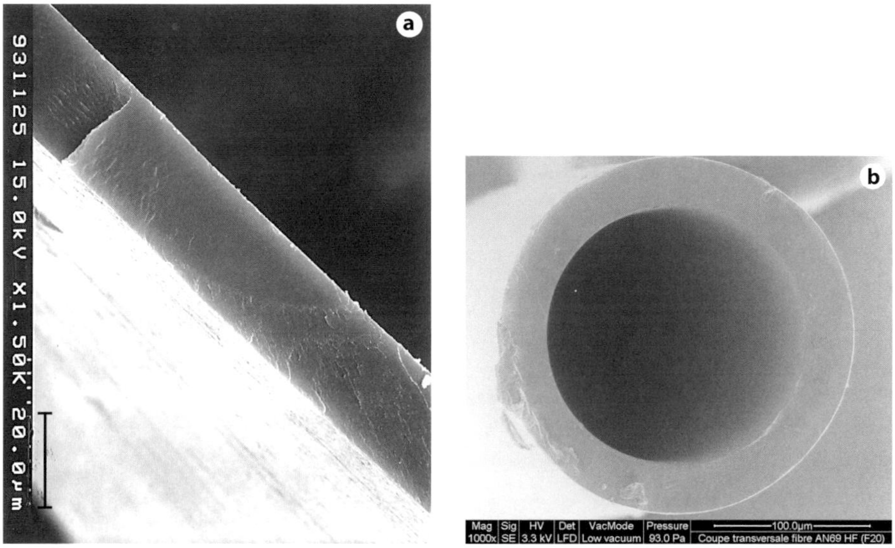

Fig. 2. SEM pictures of (**a**) AN69 flat sheet and (**b**) AN69 hollow fiber.

hydrophilic by nature because the sulfonate groups, present in large numbers, attract water and create the hydrogel structure which is important for the diffusive and hydraulic permeability [4].

The performance of a membrane stems not only from the nature of the polymer but also from the structure, which in turn is determined by the technology of the manufacturing process. A dedicated manufacturing process has been developed for AN69 based on high temperature spinning and the use of nitrogen, an inert gas, as center medium when hollow fibers are produced. The polymer nature and the specific spinning process jointly result in a symmetrical, homogeneous, hydrogel structure as shown by the SEM picture (fig. 2).

The AN69 membrane was first produced as flat sheet and since 1980 also as hollow fibers. Continuous development of the membrane has been applied in terms of thickness and internal diameter leading to improved performance. The dialyzer manufacturing process was modified in the 1980s to allow sterilization by γ-radiation instead of ethylene oxide. In response to the appearance of new

Table 1. Continuous innovative process for optimized adsorption properties

	Native AN69 flat sheet in 1972 hollow fiber in 1980	AN69 ST flat sheet in 1998 hollow fiber in 2000	HeprAN hollow fiber in 2008
Development steps	Electronegative membrane	Treatment with cationic polymer to neutralize surface charge	Further treatment with cationic polymer and heparin grafting on internal surface
Interaction with low-molecular-weight proteins	Adsorption in the membrane bulk through electrostatic interaction with negative sulfonic groups		
Interaction with high-molecular-weight proteins		Inhibition of adsorption due to surface electroneutralization	
Interaction with heparin		Adsorption through interaction with internal positive cationic groups	Grafting on internal surface
Interaction with antithrombin III		Specific adsorption by binding to heparin coating	
Interaction with bacterial derivatives endotoxin, lipid A			Adsorption through electropositive external surface

technology and new therapeutic requirements, the original AN69 membrane has been continuously modified to meet the needs of contemporary dialysis (table 1).

Membrane Adsorption – A Unique Property of AN69

Diffusion and convection are the basic transport mechanisms for solute removal in dialysis. However, with time it has become clear that adding adsorption could have major impact on removal of the large group of medium-sized uremic toxins, including protein-bound retention products. These solutes have a number of immune-depressing characteristics but are today poorly removed by contemporary dialysis membranes and modes [5].

Plasmatic substances can be adsorbed either on the surface of the membrane or throughout the membrane matrix. Surface adsorption applies mainly to high-molecular-weight proteins, e.g. albumin, which are too large to permeate the structure. It often leads to declining permeability through blocking of the pores but can also cause significant albumin loss and coagulation activation. Smaller molecules, e.g. low-/medium-molecular weight proteins, which can diffuse within the membrane structure, are adsorbed throughout the bulk of the membrane, and usually have little impact on permeability. Most interactions between plasma proteins and membranes are hydrophobic or electrostatic in nature and thus unspecific.

In the AN69 membrane the microstructure and the chemical composition offer a unique context for bulk adsorption of low-molecular-weight proteins, the high water content of the hydrogel making the polymer chains easily accessible. The ionic characteristic of the membrane material through its sulfonate groups provides specificity for basic proteins, i.e. proteins with isoelectric point >7, e.g. many inflammatory mediators. Proteins having basic residues on the surface can also be specifically adsorbed. Because the sulfonate groups are distributed throughout the membrane structure of the AN69 membrane, surface adsorption and membrane plugging are negligible and the performance remains stable over time.

The highly specific adsorptive properties – limited on the surface and favored in the membrane structure with high specificity for medium-sized proteins with basic properties – distinguish AN69 from other synthetic high-flux membranes as well as from other so-called adsorptive membranes in the field of dialysis.

The World's First Biocompatible Membrane

During the 1980s the concept of biocompatibility emerged and spread in the dialysis world, characterizing the biological interactions occurring in blood upon contact with a foreign material and finding that a number of undesirable reactions take place during the dialysis session. Membrane-induced complement activation was used to quantify the degree of biocompatibility of different membranes and formation of the mediators of the complement cascade was documented. During dialysis with AN69, only negligible amounts of mediators such as C3a, C5a, TCC and factor D reach the bloodstream. Numerous studies rapidly established AN69 as a reference in this respect in comparison to other membranes [6, 7]. The superior biocompatibility of AN69 stems from the unique adsorptive capacity for the anaphylatoxic and inflammatory complement factors [8–10]. Other markers of biocompatibility used to rank dialysis membranes, such as release of elastase from activated granulocytes [11], loss of platelets due to adhesion to the membrane surface [12], platelet activation leading to release of β-thromboglobulin [13] and undesirable cell activation [14] all confirm the preference for AN69.

The biocompatibility of a dialysis membrane has also been shown to affect protein metabolism. A study in healthy humans shows that blood contact with the membrane has a catabolic effect, causing efflux of amino acids from muscle tissue, when a bioincompatible membrane is used, whereas exposure to AN69 has no such effect [15]. Considering the common occurrence of malnutrition and inflammation among dialysis patients, this finding further supports the use of biocompatible dialysis membranes [16].

The International Cooperative Biocompatibility Study from the early 1990s compared seven different dialyzers and ranked AN69 as 'the most biocompatible membrane and one of those allowing the best clinical tolerance' [17]. Improved survival of patients treated exclusively with AN69 was shown in retrospective analyses [18].

With time new markers of biocompatibility have appeared, one of the most recent being monocyte chemoattractant protein (MCP-1). It is of medium size (16.3 kDa), present in plasma at very low concentration and involved in atherosclerosis. Removal of MCP-1 can only be achieved through specific adsorption and the molecule has been shown to have great affinity for the HeprAN membrane, the latest version of the AN69 [19].

Removal of a New Uremic Toxin – β_2-Microglobulin

Chronic arthropathy was a well-known long-term complication of dialysis therapy long before it was discovered that the osteoarticular deposits are of amyloid nature and the major constituent is β_2-microglobulin (β_2M) [20]. This 12,000-Da molecule has been added to the list of uremic retention products and the kinetics for its removal from blood were studied. The plasma levels of β_2M in anuric dialysis patients are often 30–40 times higher than normal and can only be lowered when dialysis is performed with highly permeable membranes. In addition, β_2M can be removed by adsorption and especially so to the AN69 membrane in which the basic residues on the protein surface are specifically attracted to the negatively charged sulfonate groups in the membrane. Through combined transport and adsorption the AN69 membrane was found to provide the largest total removal of β_2M from blood when compared to other high-flux membranes [21]. Although the plasma concentration of β_2M cannot be reduced to normal levels in dialysis patients, numerous publications show a clinical benefit of maximum removal and reduction. Significant risk reduction for carpal tunnel syndrome and bone cysts has been documented in patients treated with AN69 filters by several studies [22, 23].

Avoiding Contact Phase Activation

In the 1990s a new type of hypersensitivity reaction appeared among dialysis patients, rare and of varying severity but still disturbing. Further analysis showed that it could be associated with elevated levels of bradykinin indicating activation of the kallikrein-kinase system. After thorough investigations it appeared that the combined use of the AN69 membrane and ACE inhibitors, at the time a novel group of antihypertensive drugs, can lead to these reactions. The negatively charged membrane triggered activation of factor XII which via several steps resulted in formation of bradykinin, the normal breakdown of which was prevented by the drug-induced inhibition of the converting enzyme [24].

The demand for a modification of the AN69 membrane to allow continued safe use for all patients was urgent. The membrane engineers succeeded to reduce the surface adsorption properties for high-molecular-weight proteins, such as fibrinogen, kininogen and factor XII, without affecting the bulk adsorption of low-/medium-sized proteins. This was achieved by neutralizing the surface in contact with blood by ionic grafting of a polycationic polymer, polyethyleneimine (PEI). The result was validated by showing a corresponding reduction of the surface electrical potential, the ζ potential [25] and the absence of contact phase activation [24]. The modified membrane has been named AN69ST, with ST standing for surface treated.

Heparin Coating and Grafting Can Provide Heparin-Free Dialysis

The reduced electronegativity of the membrane surface in the AN69ST membrane allows binding of heparin when primed with a heparin solution prior to use. This opens the possibility for significant reduction of the systemic dose of heparin and even makes heparin-free dialysis possible for patients with high risk of bleeding [26, 27].

To facilitate the preparation of the dialyzer it was desirable to eliminate the heparin priming in the dialysis unit and integrate this step in the manufacturing of the dialyzer. This could be realized in 2008 by grafting heparin to the AN69ST membrane. New technology enabled unfractionated heparin to be grafted to the membrane directly during the manufacturing process, and a reproducible amount of heparin is bound to the membrane with high chemical and biological stability [28]. According to the European medical device directive filters with the new HeprAN membrane, Evodial, represent the first class III dialyzers, i.e. combined medical device and drug. For approval in this category the design of the HeprAN membrane, particularly the grafting stability, reproducibility and the industrial process and traceability of the heparin used, have been validated through CE marking procedure. The heparin grafted onto the membrane has specific affinity for antithrombin III which is adsorbed on the surface and allows neutralization of thrombin through thrombin-antithrombin in a reversible process. A clinical study showed rapid decline of factor anti-Xa during dialysis with Evodial in patients with elevated levels at start and as a consequence significantly reduced need for systemic heparinization [29].

The heparin grafting to the inner surface of the membrane requires intensified treatment with the polycationic polymer PEI, and this has opened up the possibility to treat also the outer surface. The result is considerably increased adsorption capacity on those parts of the membrane exposed to dialysis fluid. Bacterial products, e.g. endotoxin and Lipid A are negatively charged and thus preferentially adsorbed. This additional characteristic of the Evodial dialyzers makes them a safe choice for contemporary high-flux dialysis, in which the non-sterile dialysis fluid reaches the bloodstream after reverse filtration and backdiffusion through the membrane of the dialyzer.

A Membrane for Acute Renal Failure and Sepsis

Filters with AN69 membrane have been used to treat acute renal failure since the early days, often with excellent outcome [30] and are still the preferred choice for many nephrologists and intensivists [31]. To treat severe inflammatory conditions, sepsis or septic shock, it is believed to be necessary to reduce the level of inflammatory mediators. Many water-soluble mediators with pro- and anti-inflammatory action have medium/high molecular weight (TNF-α 17 kDa, IL-6 26 kDa, IL-10 30 kDa) and are thus poorly removed by dialysis even when high-flux membranes and convective transport is applied. It has been hypothesized that adding adsorption to the dialytic transport mechanisms could enhance the removal, especially with a membrane like AN69ST which has adsorptive properties in addition to being highly permeable and biocompatible. In fact, hemofiltration with AN69 has been shown constantly and efficiently remove cytokines from blood, mainly by adsorption to the membrane matrix of the hemofilter [32]. Continuous veno-venous hemofiltration using AN69 is reported to be effective in removing many plasma cytokines, improving immune dysfunction and increasing monocyte HLA-DR expression [33]. Additionally, it was recently demonstrated that the high mobility group box 1 protein, HMGB1, a 30-kDa alarmin which plays an important role in sepsis, can be significantly removed using AN69ST in vitro [34].

Still a Unique High Permeability Membrane for Chronic and Acute Renal Patients

A wide range of high permeability dialysis membranes are available today and it is noteworthy that modern versions of the first membrane with this characteristic are still the preferred choice for many patients. Since its creation in the early 1970s, the AN69 membrane has evolved to meet the requirements and challenges of dialysis therapy. Still the basic characteristics of high permeability to fluid and to a wide range of relevant uremic retention products combined with excellent biocompatibility, whether measured by traditional or novel indicators, have remained the hallmark of the membrane. The unique adsorptive capacity, adding to the total removal of targeted solutes such as β_2M, has been the base for future development. The latest version of AN69, the HeprAN membrane, has heparin grafting on the inner surface and enhanced adsorption of bacterial products on the outer surface. Modern versions of AN69 are today used in hemodialysis and contemporary modes of convective therapies for a large number of chronic as well as acute renal patients around the world [35, 36].

References

1 Man NK, Granger A, Rondon-Nucete M, Zingraff J, Jungers P, Sausse A, Funck-Brentano JL: One year follow-up of short dialysis with a membrane highly permeable to middle molecules. Proc EDTA. 1973;10:236–246.

2 Babb AL, Popovich RP, Christopher TG, Scribner BH: The genesis of the square meter-hour hypothesis. Trans. ASAIO 1971;17:81–91.

3 Chanard J, Brunois JP, Melin JP, Lavaud S, Toupance O: Long-term results of dialysis therapy with a highly permeable membrane. Artif Organs 1982;6:261–266.

4 Cohen-Addad JP, Brunelet A, Bazile JP, Buda A, Thomas M: Acrylonitrile-sodium methallylsulfonate copolymer. DSC approach to membrane porosity of foam and hollow fibers. Biomaterials 2003;24:173–179.

5 Vanholder R, Argiles A, Baurmeister U, Brunet P, Clark W, Cohen G, De Deyn PP, Deppisch R, Descamps-Latscha B, Henle T, Joerres A, Massy ZA, Rodriguez M, Stegmayr B, Stenvinkel P, Wratten ML: Uremic toxicity: present state of the art. Int J Artif Organs 2001;24:695–725.

6 Foret M, Hachache T, Meftahi H, Milongo R, Kuentz F, Christollet M, Alibeu C, Cordonnier DJ: The long-term evaluation of the biocompatibility of nine different haemodialysis membranes. Life Support Syst 1987;5:203–206.

7 Martin-Malo A, Castillo D, Castro M, Perez R, Rios A, Jaraba M, Aljama P: Biocompatibility of dialysis membranes; a comparative study. Nephrol Dial Transplant 1991;6(suppl 2):55–58.

8 Cheung AK, Chenoweth DE, Otsuka D, Henderson LW: Compartmental distribution of complement activation products in artificial kidneys. Kidney Int 1986;30:74–80.

9 Kandus A, Ponikvar R, Drinovec J, Kladnik S, Ivanovich P: Anaphylatoxins C3a and C5a adsorption on acrylonitrile membrane of hollow-fiber and plate dialyzer – an in vivo study. Int J Artif Organs 1990;13:176–180.

10 Pascual M, Schifferli JA: Adsorption of complement factor D by polyacrylonitrile dialysis membranes. Kidney Int 1993;43:903–911.

11 Hoerl WH, Steinhauer HB, Schollmeyer P: Plasma levels of granulocyte elastase during hemodialysis: effects of different dialyzer membranes. Kidney Int 1985;28:791–796.

12 Docci D, Turci F, Del Vecchio C, Bilancioni R, Cenciotti L, Pretolani E: Hemodialysis-associated platelet loss: study of the relative contribution of dialyzer membrane composition and geometry. Int J Artif Organs 1984;7:337–340.

13 Verbeelen D, Jochmans K, Herman AG, Van der Niepen P, Sennesael J, De Waele M: Evaluation of platelets and hemostasis during hemodialysis with six different membranes. Nephron 1991;59:567–572.

14 Descamps-Latscha B, Herbelin A, Nguyen AT, De Groote D, Chauveau P, Verger C, Jungers P, Zingraff J: Soluble CD23 as an effector of immune dysregulation in chronic uremia and dialysis. Kidney Int 1993;43:878–884.
15 Gutierrez A, Alvestrand A, Wahren J, Bergstroem J: Effect of in vivo contact between blood and dialysis membranes on protein catabolism in humans. Kidney Int 1990;38:487–494.
16 Stenvinkel P: Inflammatory and atherosclerotic interactions in the depleted uremic patient. Blood Purif 2001;19:53–61.
17 Levin NW, Zasuwa G: Relationship between dialyser type and signs and symptoms. Nephrol Dial Transplant 1993;8(suppl.2):30–39.
18 Chandran PKG, Liggett R, Kirkpatrick B: Patient survival on PAN/AN69 membrane hemodialysis: a ten-year analysis. J Am Soc Nephrol 1993;4:1199–1204.
19 Morena M, Jaussent I, Chalabi L, Bargnoux AS, Dupuy AM, Badiou S, Rakic C, Thomas M, Canaud B, Cristol JP: Biocompatibility of heparin-grafted hemodialysis membranes: impact on monocyte chemoattractant protein-1 circulating level and oxidative status. Hemodial Int 2010;14:403–410.
20 Gejyo F, Yamada T, Odani S, Nakagawa Y, Arakawa M, Kunitomo T, Kataoka H, Suzuki M, Hirasawa Y, Shirahama T, Cohen AS, Schmid K: A new form of amyloid protein associated with chronic hemodialysis was identified as β_2-microglobulin. Biochem Biophys Res Commun 1985;129:701–706.
21 Floege J, Granolleras C, Deschodt G, Heck M, Baudin G, Branger B, Tournier O, Reinhard B, Eisenbach GM, Smeby LC, Koch KM, Shaldon S: High-flux synthetic versus cellulosic membranes for β_2-microglobulin removal during hemodialysis, hemodiafiltration and hemofiltration. Nephrol Dial Transplant 1989;7:653–657.
22 Chanard J, Bindi P, Lavaud S, Toupance O, Maheut H, Lacour F: Carpal tunnel syndrome and type of dialysis membrane. BMJ 1989;298:867–868.
23 Van Ypersele De Strihou C, Jadoul M, Malghem J, Maldague B, Jamart J, The Working Party on Dialysis Amyloidosis: Effect of dialysis membrane and patient's age on signs of dialysis related amyloidosis. Kidney Int 1991;39:1012–1019.
24 Desormeaux A, Moreau ME, Lepage Y, Chanard J, Adam A: The effect of electronegativity and angiotensin-converting enzyme inhibition on the kinin-forming capacity of polyacrylonitrile dialysis membranes. Biomaterials 2008;29:1139–1146.
25 Renaux JL, Thomas M, Crost T, Loughraieb N, Vantard G: Activation of the kallikrein-kinin system in hemodialysis: role of membrane electronegativity, blood dilution, and pH. Kidney Int 1999;55:1097–1103.
26 Lavaud S, Paris B, Maheut H, Randoux C, Renaux JL, Rieu P, Chanard J: Assessment of the heparin-binding AN69ST hemodialysis membrane. 2. Clinical studies without heparin administration. ASAIO J 2005;51:348–351.
27 Chanard J, Lavaud S, Maheut H, Kazes I, Vitry F, Rieu P: The clinical evaluation of low-dose heparin in haemodialysis: a prospective study using the heparin-coated AN69ST membrane. Nephrol Dial Transplant 2008;23:2003–2009.
28 Chanard J, Karaaslan H, Lavaud S, Rieu P, Arkouche W, Cardoso J, Tielemans C: A new synthetic heparinized hemodialyzer membrane. J Am Soc Nephrol 2008;19:F-PO1580.
29 Kessler M, Cao Huu T, Gutierrez A, Coudert-Krier M-J, Kielstein JT, Gangemi C, Galland R, Moussion-Schott F: Heparin-grafted dialysis membrane permits minimal systemic anticoagulation and a lower anti-Xa level at treatment end. J Am Soc Nephrol 2010;21:8–9A.
30 Schiffl H, Lang SM, Koenig A, Strasser T, Haider MC, Held E: Biocompatible membranes in acute renal failure: prospective case-controlled study. Lancet 1994;344:570–572.
31 The RENAL Replacement Therapy Study Investigators: Intensity of continuous renal-replacement therapy in critically ill patients. N Engl J Med 2009;361:1627–1638.

32 De Vriese AS, Colardyn FA, Philippe JJ, Vanholder RC, De Sutter JH, Lameire NH: Cytokine removal during continuous hemofiltration in septic patients. J Am Soc Nephrol 1999;10:846–853.
33 Peng Z, Pai P, Hong-Bao L, Rong L, Han-Min W, Chen H: The impact of continuous veno-venous hemofiltration on plasma cytokines and monocyte human leukocyte antigen-DR expression in septic patients. Cytokine 2010;50:186–191.
34 Yumoto M, Nishida O, Moriyama K, Shimomura Y, Nakamura N, Kuriyama N, Hara Y, Yamada S, Miyasho T: In vitro evaluation of HMGB1 removal with various membranes for continuous hemofiltration. Crit Care 2011;15(suppl 1):S41.
35 Potier J: Feasibility between AN69 and hemodiafiltration online (in French). Nephrol Ther 2010;6:21–27.
36 Rimmele T, Kellum JA: Clinical review: blood purification for sepsis. Crit Care 2011;15:205–214.

Ingrid Ledebo, PhD
Gambro R&D
Box 10101, SE 220 20 Lund (Sweden)
Tel. +46 46 169 176
E-Mail ingrid.ledebo@gambro.com

Saito A, Kawanishi H, Yamashita AC, Mineshima M (eds): High-Performance Membrane Dialyzers.
Contrib Nephrol. Basel, Karger, 2011, vol 173, pp 130–136

Polyethersulfone as a High-Performance Membrane

Detlef H. Krieter[a] · Horst-Dieter Lemke[b]

[a]University Hospital Würzburg, Department of Medicine, Division of Nephrology and
[b]Membrana GmbH, Research & Development, Wuppertal, Germany

Abstract

Polyethersulfone as base material has proven its suitability for synthetic dialysis membranes since more than one decade. Recently, a new generation of high-performance polyethersulfone membranes has been introduced, which are the result of an advanced spinning process. They are characterized by an improved permselectivity due to a more homogenous and dense pore size distribution. These innovative membranes achieve an outstanding middle molecule removal at low albumin loss and have best biocompatibility characteristics. Provided that the albumin permeability is low, the pyrogen retention capability is on a par with the best references. Overall, polyethersulfone high-performance membranes are highly efficient, biocompatible, safe and suited for all current dialysis procedures.

During the last years, some new synthetic dialysis membranes have been introduced, which ideally combine best biocompatibility characteristics with excellent toxin removal due to improved permselectivity. Like most synthetic membranes, this new class of high-performance membranes consists of a blend of hydrophobic base polymers, which favorably determines biocompatibility, and hydrophilic components to improve transmembrane solute passage. The chemical composition, i.e. the base polymer and the ratio of base polymer and copolymer, is particularly important for the pore morphology and pore size distribution of a membrane, but also the sophisticated spinning process determines the sieving characteristics. While polyvinylpyrrolidone is widely used as the hydrophilic component, polysulfone and polyethersulfone have become the dominating polymers for high-performance membrane composition.

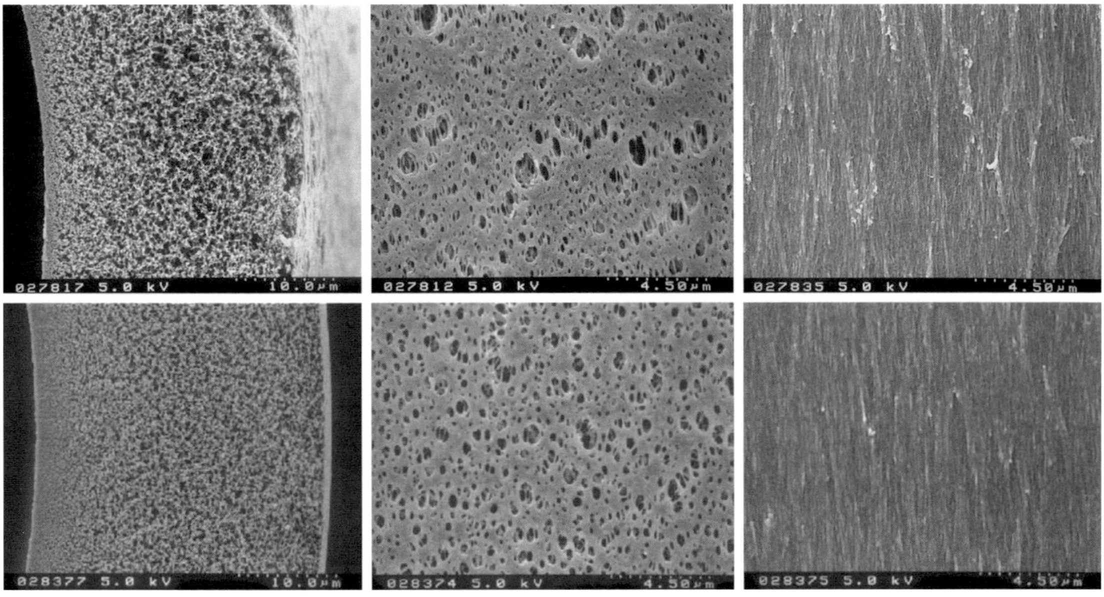

Fig. 1. Electron microscopic views of first-generation (Diapes® HF800, upper row) and second-generation (Purema® H, lower row) PES membranes: cross section (left), outer (middle) and inner surface (right) with thicker separation layer (left pair) and more even pore size distribution (middle pair) (figures courtesy of Membrana GmbH, Germany).

Evolution of Polyethersulfone High-Performance Membranes

Polyethersulfone (synonymous: polyarylethersulfone) as base polymer for a synthetic high-flux dialysis membrane was introduced in 2000 [1]. This Diapes® HF800-labeled, microreticular membrane (Membrana GmbH, Wuppertal, Germany) differs from chemically similar polysulfone membranes in its three-layer wall structure with lower wall diameter (30 μm) (fig. 1). It can be used for hemodialysis and more convective therapy forms, i.e. hemofiltration and hemodiafiltration.

As a further development of Diapes® HF800, which already was a very efficient membrane in terms of middle molecule permeability, the Purema® H membrane (Membrana GmbH) was introduced in 2007 [2]. The product of a modified spinning process, which is characterized by specific addition of negatively charged polyelectrolytes to the inner separating layer of the membrane, Purema® H has a similar water flux but a more homogenous and dense pore size distribution (table 1; fig. 1) compared to its polyethersulfone precursor [2]. The modification of the pore morphology results in a significantly steeper sieving curve for low-molecular-weight proteins (table 1) complying with the engineering target of minimum albumin permeability at maximum permeability for

Table 1. In vitro characteristics of the high-flux polyethersulfone membranes Diapes® HF800 and Purema®H. Table modified from Krieter et al. [2]

	High-flux polyethersulfone	
	Purema® H	Diapes® HF800
Membrane material	polyethersulfone-polyvinylpyrrolidone blend	polyethersulfone-polyvinylpyrrolidone blend
Wall structure	asymmetric, two-layer	asymmetric, three-layer
Fiber diameter, μm	200	200
Wall diameter, μm	30	30
Sieving coefficient		
Cytochrome C (12,400 Da)	0.95 ± 0.04*	0.60 ± 0.05
Albumin (67,000 Da)	0.001 ± 0.001*	0.005 ± 0.002
KUF, mL/h • m² • mm Hg	85.3 ± 11.7	82.6 ± 11.5

* p < 0.001 vs. Diapes® HF800.

low-molecular-weight proteins smaller than albumin [2]. The same is reflected by the pore size distribution calculated from sieving coefficients showing that the narrow size distribution leads to a shift of the mean pore size towards higher values enabling better passage of low-molecular-weight proteins and at the same time a reduction in the number of pores large enough to allow a loss of essential proteins and thus low albumin loss (fig. 2).

Another new-generation polyethersulfone membrane manufactured by application of advanced spinning procedures to produce uniformly sized, larger but homogenously distributed pores with a sharp cut-off is the recently introduced Polynephron™ membrane (Nipro Corp., Osaka, Japan) [3].

Effect of Polyethersulfone Membrane Modification on Clinical Performance

In a first prospective in vitro and clinical study investigating dialysis membrane performance during hemodialysis, Purema® H was compared to one of the most efficient high-flux polysulfone membranes (Helixone®), for which the application of nanotechnological principles during fabrication is claimed [4]. A much higher removal of low-molecular-weight proteins was verified for Purema® H. In a 4-hour treatment with standardized operational conditions, the reduction ratio of the prototypical middle molecular surrogate parameter β_2-microglobulin (11,800 Da) was 9.2% higher (72.3 ± 5 vs. 66.2 ± 6.1%; $p < 0.001$) [2]. With increasing molecular weight of the tested solute, the difference in the reduction ratio favoring Purema® H further increased being 124.8% higher for

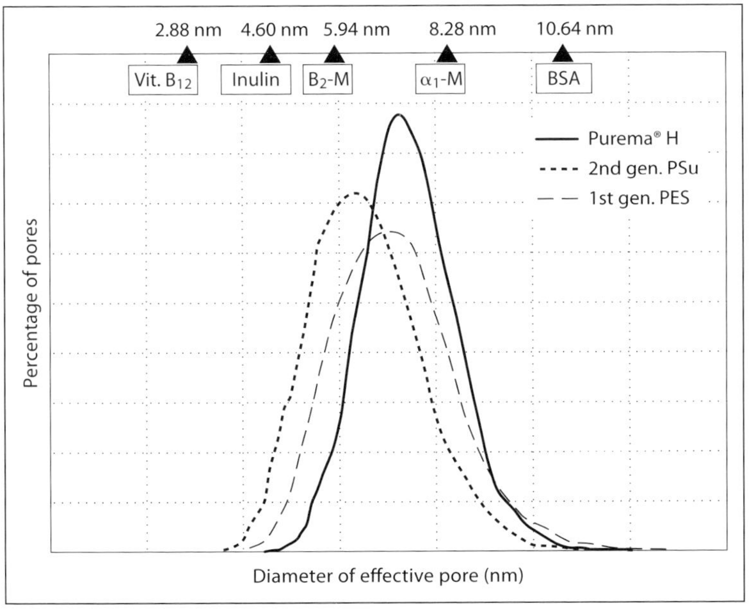

Fig. 2. Pore size distribution of second-generation PES membrane Purema® H compared to modern synthetic membranes calculated from sieving coefficients (figure courtesy of Membrana GmbH, Germany). *Vit.* B_{12} = Vitamin B_{12}; α_1*-M* = α_1-microglobulin; *BSA* = bovine serum albumin; *2nd gen. PSU* = second-generation polysulfone; *1st gen. PES* = first-generation polyethersulfone.

myoglobin (17,600 Da) compared to Helixone® (51.7 ± 7.3 vs. 23 ± 10.4%; $p < 0.001$), although the albumin loss into dialysate averaged low at only 0.53 ± 0.17 g per session [2]. Moreover, Purema® H led to significantly less pronounced leukopenia and C5a generation [2], the acknowledged key surrogate parameters of hemocompatibility. This observation was attributed to an also better removal of the middle molecular complement fragments rather than to the chemical properties of the dialysis membranes [2].

The order of magnitude of low-molecular-weight protein removal determined during hemodialysis with the polyethersulfone membrane Purema® H had previously rather been observed in more convective therapy forms, such as online postdilution hemodiafiltration [5]. Therefore, it appeared to be obvious to verify this assumption in a prospective clinical setting. Consequently, the treatment efficacy of Purema® H in hemodialysis was compared to that of high-efficiency online postdilution hemodiafiltration with two conventional synthetic high-flux membranes, namely polysulfone and Polyamix®, which are widely used for this therapy mode [6]. For most of the parameters (clearances, reduction ratios) in the range of small solutes (urea, creatinine, phosphate) and low-molecular-weight proteins (cystatin C, retinol-binding protein) no differences between the treatment modes could be determined [6]. Compared to hemodiafiltration with Polyamix®, even a significantly higher reduction ratio of myoglobin was achieved with Purema® H in hemodialysis [6]. Only the β_2-microglobulin reduction ratio of Purema® H was slightly lower versus hemodiafiltration with polysulfone (69 ± 5 vs. 73 ± 5%; $p = 0.007$) [6]. The finding of a low-molecular-weight protein removal in simple hemodialysis matching that of online hemodiafiltration is particularly remarkable since it was not a trade-off tribute to decreased membrane selectivity as the albumin loss of Purema® H was rather low [6]. In the past, a much higher albumin loss had to be accepted to realize a comparable hemodialysis treatment efficacy as a consequence of inferior dialysis membrane permselectivity [7, 8].

Polyethersulfone Membranes for Convective Treatment Procedures

It is clear that hemodialysis is not suited to fully exploit the low-molecular-weight protein removal capacity of any given high-flux dialysis membrane. However, increasing convection by hemofiltration or hemodiafiltration bears the risk of excessive albumin loss with potentially harmful consequences for the patient [9]. Both the original Purema® H and a more permeable variant named Purema® H^+ can safely be used in high-efficiency postdilution online hemodiafiltration. In this treatment mode, extremely high mean β_2-microglobulin reduction ratios of 78% have been achieved with both types, while the albumin loss did not pass 1.5 g per session [10].

In a prospective study versus the first-generation Diapes® HF800 membrane, similar results on β_2-microglobulin removal were obtained for the Polynephron™ membrane in pre- and postdilution online hemodiafiltration [3]. Being already slightly below 2 g in the hemodialysis mode, the albumin loss of Polynephron™ averaged at about 4 g in postdilution hemodiafiltration [3].

Permselectivity as a Key for Pyrogen Retention

The albumin permeability of a dialysis membrane seems to be not only a measure for the loss of an essential protein [9], but it may also indicate the pyrogen retention capability of a synthetic high-flux membrane. In recent ex vivo recirculation experiments comparing five different European high-flux dialyzers and 14 Japanese dialyzers classified type 4 and 5 according to the Japanese reimbursement system, a strong correlation ($r = 0.863$, $p < 0.0001$) between albumin permeability and cytokine induction in donor blood, as a measure of pyrogen retention, was demonstrated [11]. Confirming a previous study on pyrogen retention [12], Purema® H together with two other synthetic high-flux membranes (one polyethersulfone and one polysulfone membrane not specified) proved particularly low passage of cytokine-inducing substances indicating its safety in this regard [11]. Such test results are currently not yet available for the Polynephron™ membrane.

Conclusion

Polyethersulfone as base material has proven its suitability for high-performance synthetic dialysis membranes for more than one decade. The most recent generation of polyethersulfone membranes exhibits best biocompatibility characteristics and excellent low-molecular-weight protein removal due to an outstanding permselectivity. Provided that the albumin permeability is low, the pyrogen retention capability is on a par with the best references. Overall, polyethersulfone high-performance membranes are highly efficient, biocompatible, safe and suited for all current dialysis procedures.

References

1 Gerdemann A, Lemke HD, Nothdurft A, Heidland A, Münch G, Bahner U, Schinzel R: Low-molecular but not high-molecular advanced glycation end products are removed by high-flux dialysis. Clin Nephrol 2000;54:276–283.

2 Krieter DH, Morgenroth A, Barasinski A, Lemke HD, Schuster O, von Harten B, Wanner C: Effects of a polyelectrolyte additive on the selective dialysis membrane permeability for low-molecular-weight proteins. Nephrol Dial Transplant 2007;22:491–499.

3 Meert N, Eloot S, Schepers E, Lemke HD, Dhondt A, Glorieux G, Van Landschoot M, Waterloos MA, Vanholder R: Comparison of removal capacity of two consecutive generations of high-flux dialysers during different treatment modalities. Nephrol Dial Transplant DOI: 10.1093/ndt/gfq803.

4 Ronco C, Bowry S: Nanoscale modulation of the pore dimensions, size distribution and structure of a new polysulfone based high-flux dialysis membrane. Int J Artif Organs 2001, 24:726–735.

5 Lornoy W, Becaus I, Billiouw JM, et al: On-line haemodiafiltration. Remarkable removal of β_2-microglobulin. Long-term clinical observations. Nephrol Dial Transplant 2000;15(suppl 1):49–54.

6 Krieter DH, Hunn E, Morgenroth A, Lemke HD, Wanner C: Matching efficacy of online hemodiafiltration in simple hemodialysis mode. Artif Organs 2008;32:903–909.

7 Lucchi L, Fiore GB, Guadagni G, Perrone S, Malaguti V, Caruso F, Fumero R, Albertazzi A: Clinical evaluation of internal hemodiafiltration: diffusive-convective technique performed with internal filtration enhanced high-flux dialyzers. Int J Artif Organs 2004, 27:414–419.

8 Fujimura T, Uchi Y, Fukuda M, Miyazaki M, Uezumi S, Hiyoshi T: Development of a dialyzer with enhanced internal filtration to increase the clearance of low-molecular-weight proteins. J Artif Organs 2004, 7:149–154.

9 Krieter DH, Canaud B: High permeability of dialysis membranes: what is the limit of albumin loss? Nephrol Dial Transplant 2003;18:651–654.
10 Krieter DH, Hackl A, Rodriguez A, Chenine L, Moragues HL, Lemke HD, Wanner C, Canaud B: Protein-bound uraemic toxin removal in haemodialysis and post-dilution haemodiafiltration. Nephrol Dial Transplant 2010;25:212–218.
11 Lemke HD, Wanner C, Krieter DH: Permeability and pyrogen retention of dialysis membranes are inversely related. Kidney Dial 2010;69(suppl):59–64.
12 Krieter DH, Lemke HD, Wanner C: A new synthetic dialyzer with advanced permselectivity for enhanced low-molecular-weight protein removal. Artif Organs 2008, 32:547–554.

Detlef H. Krieter, MD
University Hospital Würzburg
Department of Medicine, Division of Nephrology
Oberdürrbacher Strasse 6, DE–97080 Würzburg (Germany)
Tel. +49 931 2013 9300, E-Mail krieter_d@medizin.uni-wuerzburg.de

Mass Transfer Mechanisms and Characteristics of High-Performance Membranes
Saito A, Kawanishi H, Yamashita AC, Mineshima M (eds): High-Performance Membrane Dialyzers.
Contrib Nephrol. Basel, Karger, 2011, vol 173, pp 137–147

Polymethylmethacrylate Membrane with a Series of Serendipity

Yoshitada Sakai

Dialysis Products Business Division, Toray Medical Co. Ltd, Urayasu, Chiba, Japan

Abstract
Forty years have passed since the polymethylmethacrylate (PMMA) membrane was first developed. This article reviews its history and explains its longevity. The membrane was developed through application of a stereocomplex phenomenon that is observed upon mixture of isotactic and syndiotactic PMMA polymers. Filtryzer™ B1 and B2 were approved in Japan in 1977. B1 was the pioneer high-performance membrane model and B2 was a model that simulated a low-flux cellulosic membrane. The development of B1 led to the development of the dialysis machine with an ultrafiltration rate (UFR)-controlling function because the UFR of B1 was too high to control using transmembrane pressure control. B1 was used not only as a dialyzer but also as a hemodiafilter by combination with a UFR controller. Biocompatibility of the dialysis membrane, complement activation and/or transient leukopenia was studied with B2. Cooperative studies between Niigata University and Toray resulted in Gejyo's finding regarding the harmfulness of β_2-microglobulin (BMG). Long-term follow-up of patients dialyzed using the BK membrane revealed that plasma BMG levels were significantly low and that the occurrence ratio of carpal tunnel syndrome was suppressed. These results were obtained by the adsorptive removal of BMG onto a PMMA membrane. Several papers have discussed new aspects in succession mainly based on clinical experiences that were not aimed at a development stage, i.e. they were kinds of serendipity. For the BK-F membrane with the largest pore size, this includes anemia and removal or modification of furancarboxylic acid, homocysteine, pentosidine and soluble CD40. For the BG membrane with a slightly anionic component, this includes pruritus and removal of free immunoglobulin light chains. Even patients' prognoses may be modified by the use of PMMA membrane. The mechanisms of these findings have been clarified bit by bit and the membrane will further open new frontiers in dialysis treatment.

Approximately 40 years have passed since the polymethylmethacrylate (PMMA) membrane was first developed as an innovative and advanced membrane. The

High-Performance Membrane (HPM) Workshop was organized in 1985 and its first annual meeting was held in March 1986. The PMMA membrane was one of the membranes presented at the beginning of the workshop. The epoch-making PMMA membrane has been used worldwide ever since. This article reviews its history and explains its longevity as a dialyzer, perpetually opening new frontiers in hemodialysis treatment.

Genesis

The PMMA membrane was developed in the Basic Research Laboratories of Toray Industries, Inc. The membrane was originally intended as a reverse osmosis (RO) membrane through the application of a stereocomplex phenomenon, which was an unfamiliar phenomenon in polymer science, peculiar to the PMMA solution. The phenomenon is observed as a thermoreversible sol/gel transition when isotactic PMMA and syndiotactic PMMA are mixed in an organic solvent.

However, the PMMA membrane's rejection on sodium chloride (NaCl) would not meet the requirements of an RO membrane, and it had low rejection levels. The PMMA membranes were evaluated not only with NaCl but also with urea as a reference organic solute to inorganic NaCl because their molecular weights are similar (58.5 and 60 Da for NaCl and urea, respectively). Vitamin B_{12} was also used as a larger evaluation molecule.

Researchers judged that use of the PMMA membrane might be more appropriate as a hemodialysis membrane [1–3] rather than an RO membrane when considering the square meter-hour hypothesis [4], a topic in the hemodialysis field at that time.

Development of the PMMA hemodialysis membrane was the first moment of serendipity.

Approval of the Filtryzer™ Family as Hemodialyzers Equipped with PMMA Membranes and Their Impact on Dialysis Treatment

The first PMMA dialyzer models were the Filtryzer B1 and B2 series, both of which were approved in 1977 in Japan and the first synthetic hollow fiber dialyzers in the world. B1 was high-flux, whereas B2 (nowadays B3) was low-flux and used a PMMA copolymer with a slightly anionic portion. The former was one of the high-performance membrane pioneers while the latter simulated the flux of the cellulosic membrane which was used as the standard dialyzer at that time.

Development of the B1 dialyzer led to the development of the dialysis machine with an ultrafiltration rate (UFR)-controlling function [5]. The UFR of the B1 was too high to appropriately control the amount of water to be removed from each patient using the transmembrane pressure-controlling mechanism used at that time. The development of a dialysis machine with a direct UFR-controlling mechanism, i.e. a machine with a flow equalizer and a UFR metering pump, was another serendipity in the dialysis field. The Filtryzer B1 was used not only as a dialyzer but also as a filter in hemodiafiltration (HDF) systems [5, 6]. These studies were pioneers in the development of the new dialysis modality, i.e. HDF.

Since the launch of Filtryzer B2 in the USA, the biocompatibilities of the different dialysis membranes with regard to complement activation and/or transient leukopenia have been studied. A massive difference between cellulosic and PMMA membranes was reported by Hakim et al. [7]. The PMMA membrane was not originally developed to have low stimulating activity on the complement system; this critical difference was obtained by serendipity.

Removal of β_2-Microglobulin

Filtryzer BK with larger pores was launched in 1984 in Japan. Toray's researchers collaborated with a Niigata University group led by Professor Arakawa and Professor Gejyo to discover harmful substances that accumulated in maintenance dialysis patients' blood. Toray devised methods to purify and concentrate these accumulated substances [8] and the Niigata University group analyzed components in the deposited amyloid. As a result of such basic endeavors, Gejyo et al. [9] finally assessed the harm of accumulated β_2-microglobulin (BMG) in patients' blood, i.e. BMG deposited as a major component of amyloid fibril in the carpal tunnel. Though Ono et al. [10] applied to the Annual Meeting of the American Society of Artificial Organs in 1986 to report the removal and dynamics in patients' body of BMG using the BK membrane, this was not accepted, presumably because it was too early to be understood correctly at that time.

In parallel to such basic research, the Filtryzer BK (more correctly, the BK-P series which was designed to optimize BMG removal) had been widely used in the dialysis facilities relating to Niigata University. Patients who were dialyzed using BK membrane were followed for 2 [11] and 8 years [12]. The study revealed that plasma BMG levels were significantly suppressed compared with those using the cellulosic low-flux membrane and that the occurrence ratios of carpal tunnel syndrome and radiolucent bone cyst were low; this was understood to be a result of BMG removal by the BK membrane [12]. Interestingly, the amount of BMG in the spent dialysate was minimal but its reduction rate in the patients' plasma was relatively high. As a result, its removal was judged as adsorptive removal of BMG onto the membrane. It was understood that the massive removal of BMG by adsorption is a result of the PMMA membrane's homogeneous structure in

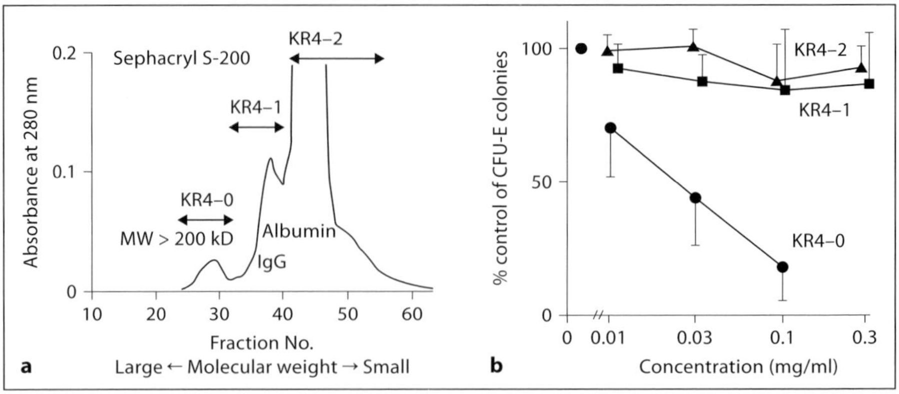

Fig. 1. a Fractionation by gel filtration of concentrated dialysate when BK-F membrane was used clinically [13]. **b** Inhibition of CFU-E colony formation by fractions from gel filtration [13]. Only KR4–0 fraction demonstrated a significant erythropoiesis-inhibiting effect dose dependently.

which the entire membrane contributes to adsorptive removal instead of permeation removal through a skin layer of polysulfone membrane.

Although HPM had been originally intended to remove larger unspecified molecules, it was reconsidered as the membrane for massive removal of BMG after the above finding by Professor Gejyo. Since then, membrane performance classification in Japan has been based on BMG removal capacity (i.e., the original 2 classes have been expanded to 5 classes).

The launch of the BK membrane and the basic research on the harmfulness of BMG led to the discovery of massive BMG removal by adsorption; this was another instance of serendipity.

Removal or Modification of Plasma Components by a Protein-Leaking PMMA Membrane

The Filtryzer BK-F, with the largest pore size among the PMMA membranes, was developed to remove accumulated components larger than BMG that may relate to long-term dialysis complications. Various investigations have proceeded using the BK-F dialyzer. A possible amelioration effect of the BK-F dialyzer on anemia has been sporadically reported and the mechanism of this effect was confirmed by Yamada et al. [13]. Figure 1 shows the main result: only the larger molecule KR4–0 suppressed colony-forming unit-erythroid (CFU-E) colony formation. Niwa et al. [14] reported removal of furancarboxylic acid by the BK-F membrane, one of the protein-bound uremic toxins. Galli et al. [15] reported that the BK-F membrane could significantly reduce

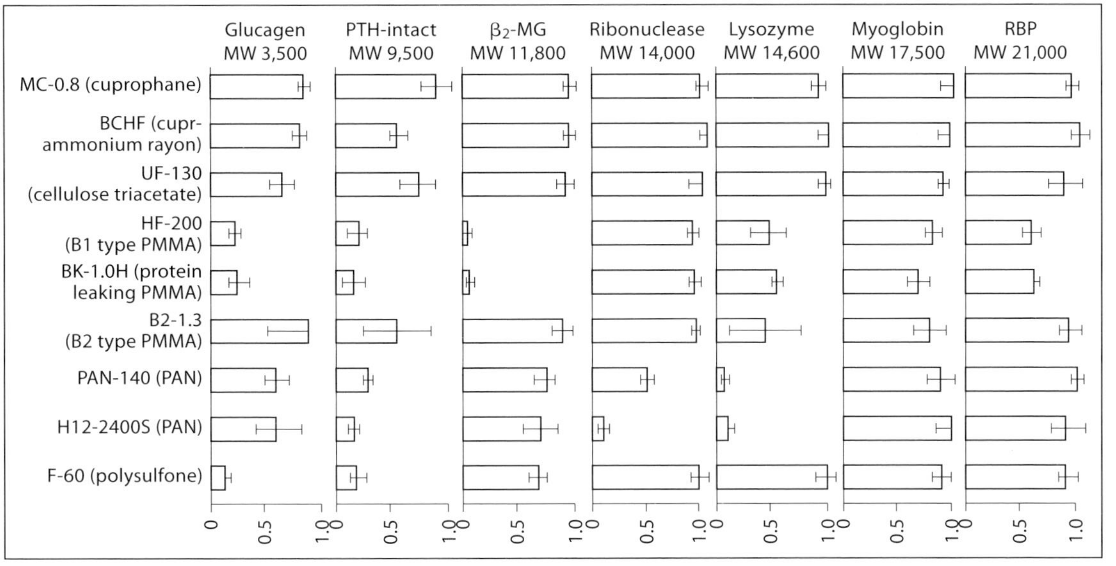

Fig. 2. Relative concentrations of low-molecular-weight proteins in dialysis patient plasma after 3 h incubation with various dialysis membranes [17].

the pre-dialysis total plasma homocysteine (Hcy) level after 3 months. Hcy is one of the protein-bound uremic toxins that is recognized as a risk factor for cardiovascular disease. They also reported that the BK-F membrane reduced the levels of total pentosidine, protein carbonyls, advanced oxidation protein product, and inflammatory cytokines (interleukin (IL)-1β, IL-6, and tumor necrosis factor-α) [16].

Removal of Various Protein Components by Adsorption

Suzuki [17] reported on the removal rate of protein components in patient plasma by various membranes in an in vitro experiment (fig. 2). BK-H and B1, which have the larger pore sizes among the PMMA membranes, remove not only BMG but also intact PTH (iPTH) as compared with other membranes. There have been successive reports on the general adsorptive removal of proteins by PMMA membranes [18–20]. Figure 3 shows Aoike's data [19], a two-dimensional electrophoresis pattern of samples from plasma of a hemodialysis patient and a normal subject. It is apparent that many protein components accumulate in patients' plasma.

Pruritus or itching is one of the long-term complications concomitant with dialysis therapy. Many hypotheses about the cause of dialysis-related pruritus have been proposed. One such hypothesis states that pruritus is

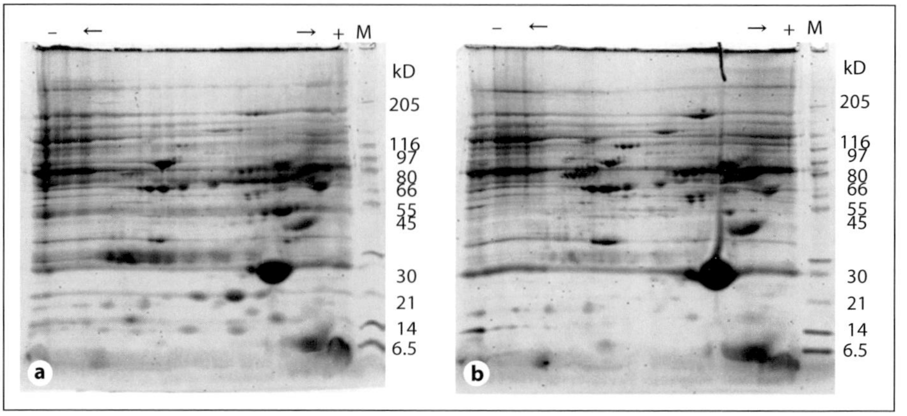

Fig. 3. Two-dimensional electrophoresis pattern of sample from plasma. M = Marker molecules. **a** Hemodialysis patient. **b** Normal subject [19].

caused by accumulation of pruritus-inducing substances. Sporadic reports had described the ameliorative effect of PMMA membranes, the Filtryzer BG in particular, on pruritus. Yamada et al. [21] studied in an in vitro system which histamine release-inducing factors, if any, could be removed using a PMMA membrane. The study showed that histamine release-inducing components whose molecular weight was assessed as 160 kDa can be removed by adsorption.

Aucella et al. [22] followed 8 patients who had been treated with low-flux synthetic membranes and were suffering from chronic itching. Their dialysis membranes were switched to the Filtryzer BG-U, and their itching strengths and durations were followed for 6 months using visual analog scale scores. The results they obtained, shown in figure 4a, indicate a decreasing itching tendency. In addition, they did not find any factors relating to the change in itching that had been hypothesized as causative factors of itching, such as effective Kt/V and iPTH. They speculated that ionic substances may be directly or indirectly adsorbed by the BG-U membrane.

Lin et al. [23] reported similar results in 30 patients with severe pruritus among 300 hemodialysis patients whose dialyzers were changed to BG-U membranes and who were then followed for 4 weeks. Pruritus severity was evaluated using a questionnaire and laboratory parameters were also pursued. The pruritus scores reduced significantly as shown in figure 4b. There were no significant differences in pre-dialysis values of BUN, Cr, BMG, Ca, phosphate, Ca-P product, iPTH, ferritin, hematocrit, hs-CRP, IL-1β, IL-2, IL-6, IL-18, TNF-α, Kt/V and BMG clearance.

The Filtryzer BG-U was not developed for such uses, hence the amelioration effect on pruritus was a kind of serendipity.

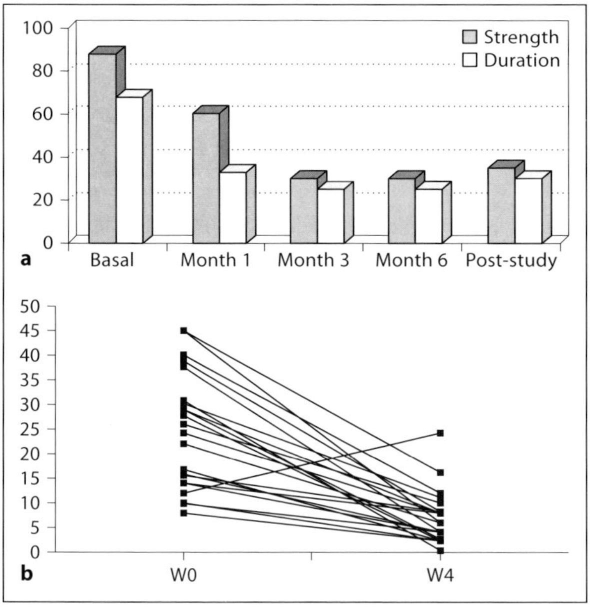

Fig. 4. Changes of pruritus of dialysis patients when BG-U membrane was used. **a** Strength and duration of self-assessed pruritus for 6 months' use of BG and 2 months after return to baseline conditions [22]. **b** Changes of pruritus score from before BG use (W0) to 4 weeks after BG use (W4) [23].

Recent Studies on the Removal or Modification of Specific Substances by PMMA Dialyzers

Several reports have described findings regarding concentration changes of specific substances, suggesting their possible clinical meaning.

Contin et al. [24] incidentally found that soluble serum CD40 (sCD40) decreased when BK-F membrane was used in their immunological study on dialysis patients. sCD40 is known to interfere with the CD40/CD154 interaction, which may then interfere with information transfer between T and B cells. They then suggested that clinically the decrease of sCD40 might lead to the improvement in the antibody seroconversion rate for anti-HBV vaccination [25].

Cohen et al. [26] studied plasma levels of free immunoglobulin light chains (FLCs) in dialysis patients. They reported that FLCs were elevated in dialysis patients, and only the PMMA membrane (speculated as BK-P) could significantly reduce the level compared to other kinds of membranes and HDF mode. Oshihara et al. [27] also investigated whether the FLCs would be reduced by the use of BG-PQ (which has the largest pore size in the BG series) for patients who had been treated by HDF with other membranes, and found that FLCs accumulated as multiple structures in the blood of hemodialysis patients and that they could be removed by adsorption to the membrane.

Other Recent Topics without Sufficient Understanding on Their Mechanism

Although the mechanism of such results has not been clarified, some reports have described other points differing from regular ones.

Masakane [28] reported that the body weights of patients whose membranes were changed from the PMMA membrane (BK-U) to the polysulfone membrane tended to decrease and that the reverse tendency was observed when the membrane was changed reversely. As such, it was concluded that the PMMA membrane is superior for maintaining body weight or muscular volume, especially in elderly patients.

Kreusser et al. [29] reported that the cumulative 5-year survival rate for dialysis patients treated with the PMMA membrane is higher than that of patients treated with the polysulfone membrane (68 vs. 54%). The representative reason for using the PMMA membrane was pruritus, thus the results remind us of the report by Pisoni et al. [30] who concluded that the pruritus/mortality relationship may be attributed to poor sleep quality.

Furthermore, statistics of the Japanese Society for Dialysis Therapy (JSDT) showed that when the prognoses of dialysis patients were compared to their dialysis membranes used under correction for basic factors (age, gender, dialysis period and underlying disease), dialysis amount, nutritional parameters and membrane surface area, those of patients treated with the PMMA membrane were significantly better [31].

Although these results individually leave some room for discussion, they are collectively heading in the same direction.

Concluding Remarks

Figure 5 summarizes the developing history, basic characteristics and the clinical findings of PMMA dialyzers which were described in this review. Although the mechanisms of some of the clinical findings have been clarified, those of others remain to be clarified.

As described before, the PMMA membrane has functioned as a pioneer in many aspects of dialysis treatment. Many components accumulate in patients' plasma (fig. 3), and many substances are speculated as uremic toxins [32]. The meaning of removal or modification of those substances are yet to be sufficiently investigated. Endeavors to open new frontiers beyond conventional viewpoints such as removal of small molecules and substances such as BMG whose harmfulness has been confirmed, or so-called biocompatibility, will be

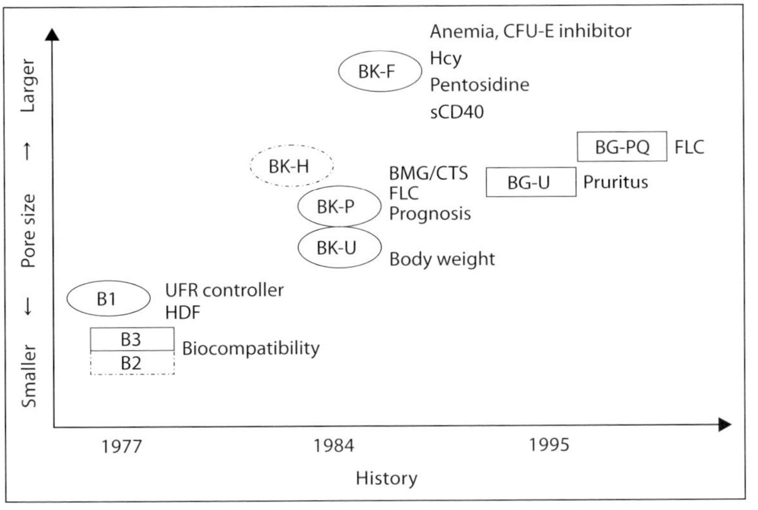

Fig. 5. Summary of this review: developing history, characteristics as membrane and clinical findings of various PMMA dialyzers. Series shown in rectangular or circular frames are slightly anionic or non-ionic membranes, respectively. B2 and BK-H series are not marketed now.

pursued. It is expected that the PMMA membrane will further contribute to such endeavors.

References

1 Sakai Y, Tanzawa H: Poly(methylmethacrylate) membranes. J Appl Polymer Sci 1978;22:1805–1815.
2 Sakai Y, Tsukamoto H, Fujii Y, Tanzawa H: Formation of poly(methylmethacrylate) membranes utilizing stereocomplex phenomenon; in Cooper AR (ed): Ultrafiltration Membranes and Applications. New York, Plenum Publishing, 1980, pp 99–107.
3 Ota K, Okazawa T, Kumagaya E, Sugino N, Mitani N, Fujii Y, Kimura M, Nagao Y, Tsukamoto H, Tanzawa H, Sakai Y: Polymethylmethacrylate capillary kidney highly permeable to middle molecules. Proc Eur Dial Transplant Assoc 1975;12:559–564.
4 Babb AL, Popovichi RP, Christopher TG, Scribner BH: The genesis of the square meter-hour hypothesis. Transact Am Soc Artif Intern Organs 1971;17:81–91.
5 Kunitomo T, Lowrie EG, O'Brien M, Lazarus JM, Gottlieb MN, Kumazawa S, Merrill JP: Performance and clinical use of a convertible hemodialysis-ultrafiltration system. Proc Dialysis Transplant Forum 1976;120–127.
6 Kunitomo T, Lowrie EG, Kumazawa S, O'Brien, Lazarus JM, Gottlieb MN, Merrill JP: Controlled ultrafiltration (UF) with hemodialysis (HD): analysis of coupling between convective and diffusive mass transfer in a new HD-UF system. Trans Am Soc Artif Intern Organs 1977;23:234–243.
7 Hakim RM, Fearon DT, Lazarus JM, Perzanowski CS: Biocompatibility of dialysis membranes: effects of chronic complement activation. Kidney Int 1982;26:194–200.

8 Kataoka H, Gejyo F, Yamada S, Kunitomo T, Arakawa M: Inhibitory effects of β_2-microglobulin on in vitro calcification of osteoblastic cells. Biochem Biophys Res Commun 1986;141:360–366.

9 Gejyo F, Yamada T, Odani S, Nakagawa Y, Arakawa M, Kunitomo T, Kataoka H, Suzuki M, Hirasawa Y, Shirahama T, Cohen AS, Schmid K: A new form of amyloid protein associated with chronic hemodialysis was identified as β_2-microglobulin. Biochem Biophys Res Commun 1985;129:701–706.

10 Ono T, Iwamoto N, Yamamoto N, Kataoka H, Yamada S, Kunitomo T: Dynamic behavior of β_2-microglobulin in chronic dialysis (HD) patients. Abstr Trans Am Soc Artif Intern Organs 1986:37.

11 Arakawa M, Niigata Research Programme for B2-M Removal Membrane: Long-term multicentre study on β_2-microglobulin removal by PMMA BK membrane. Nephrol Dial Transplant 1991(suppl 2):69–74.

12 Aoike I, Niigata Reaearch Programme for β_2-microglobulin Removal Membrane: Long-term clinical experience with PMMA membrane; in Ronco C (ed): Polymethylmethacrylate. A Flexible Membrane for a Tailored Dialysis. Basel, Karger, 1998, vol 125, pp 205–212.

13 Yamada S, Kataoka H, Kobayashi H, Ono T, Minakuchi J, Kawano Y: Identification of an erythropoietic inhibitor from the dialysate collected in the hemodialysis with PMMA membrane (BK-F) and its clinical effects; in Ronco C (ed): Polymethylmethacrylate. A Flexible Membrane for a Tailored Dialysis. Basel, Karger, 1998, vol 125, pp 159–172.

14 Niwa T, Miyazaki T, Maeda K. Removal of furancarboxylic acid, a protein-bound uremic toxin, by hemodialysis using large-pore membrane dialyzer. Jpn J Artif Organs 1995;24:694–696.

15 Galli F, Benedetti S, Buoncristiani U, Piroddi M, Conte C, Canestrari F, Buoncristiani E, Floridi A; The effect of PMMA-based protein-leaking dialyzers on plasma homocysteine levels. Kidney Int 2003;64:748–755.

16 Galli F, Benedetti S, Floridi A, Canestrari F, Piroddi M, Buoncristiani E, Buoncristiani U: Glycoxidation and inflammatory markers in patients on treatment with PMMA-based protein-leaking dialyzers. Kidney Int 2005;67:750–759.

17 Suzuki M: Recent advances of high-performance membranes for hemodialysis. Membrane 1992;17:2–11 (Japanese).

18 Birk H-W, Kistner A, Wizemann V, Schütterle: Protein adsorption by artificial membrane materials under filtration condition. Artif Organs 1995;19:411–415.

19 Aoike I: Clinical significance of protein adsorbable membranes – long-term clinical effects and analysis using a proteomic technique. Nephrol Dial Transplant 2007;22(suppl 5):v13–v19.

20 Ishikawa I, Chikazawa Y, Sato K, Nakagawa M, Imamura H, Hayama S, Yamaya H, Asaka M, Tomosugi N, Yokoyama H, Matsumoto K: Proteomic analysis of serum, outflow dialysate and adsorbed protein onto dialysis membranes (polysulfone and PMMA) during hemodialysis treatment using SELDI-TOF-MS. Nephrology 2006;26:372–380.

21 Yamada S, Sugaya H, Aoike I, Ohbayashi H, Suzuki M, Yamagishi T, Kumagai M, Okada M, Shimada H, Nakagawa Y, Kutsuwada T, Gejyo F: Isolation of mast cell degranulation factor from dialysis patients with pruritus and its removal by dialysis membranes. Kidney Dial 2003;55(suppl):167–171 (Japanese).

22 Aucella F, Vigilante M, Gesuete A, Maruccio G, Specchio A, Gesualdo L: Uraemic itching: do polymethylmethacrylate dialysis membranes play a role? Nephrol Dial Transplant 2007;22(suppl 5):v8–v12.

23 Lin HH, Liu YL, Liu JH, Chou CY, Yang YF, Kuo HL, Huang CC: Uremic pruritus, cytokines, and polymethylmethacrylate artificial kidney. Artif Organs 2008;32:468–472.

24 Contin C, Pitard V, Delmas Y, Pelletier N, Defrance T, Moreau J-F, Merville P, Déchanet-Merville J: Potential role of soluble CD40 in the humoral immune response impairment of ureamic patients. Immunology 2003;110:131–140.

25 Contin-Bordes C, Lacraz A, de Precigout V: Potential role of the soluble form of CD40 in deficient immunological function of dialysis patients: new findings of its amelioration using polymethylmethacrylate membrane. NDT Plus 2010;3(suppl 1):i20–i27.

26 Cohen G, Rudnicki M, Schmaldienst S, Hörl W-H: Effect of dialysis on serum/plasma levels of free immunoglobulin light chains in end-stage renal disease patients. Nephrol Dial Transplant 2002;17:879–883.

27 Oshihara W, Nagao H, Megano H, Arai J, Koide M, Takada M: Trial use of a polymethylmethacrylate membrane for the removal of free immunoglobulin light chains in dialysis patients. NDT Plus 2010;3(suppl 1):i3–i7.
28 Masakane I: High-quality dialysis: a lesson from the Japanese experience. NDT Plus 2010;3(suppl 1):i28–i35.
29 Kreusser W, Reiermann S, Vogelbusch G, Bartual J, Schulze-Lohoff E: Effect of different synthetic membranes on laboratory parameters and survival in chronic haemodialysis patients. NDT Plus 2010;3(suppl 1):i12–i19.
30 Pisoni RL, Wikström B, Elder SJ, Akizawa T, Asano Y, Keen ML, Saran R, Mendelssohn DC, Young EW, Port FK: Pruritus in haemodialysis patients: international results from the Dialysis Outcomes and Practice Patterns Study (DOPPS). Nephrol Dial Transplant 2006;21:3495–3505.
31 JSDT Statistical Committee: An overview of regular dialysis treatment in Japan as of December 31, 2009. Tokyo, JSDT, 2010, pp 73–74.
32 Vanholder R, Smet RD, Glorieux G, et al: Review on uremic toxins: classification, concentration, and interindividual variability. Kidney Int 2003;63:1934–1943.

Yoshitada Sakai
Dialysis Products Business Division, Toray Medical Co. Ltd
8-1, Mihama 1-chome, Urayasu, Chiba 279-8555 (Japan)
Tel. +81 47 700 7537
E-Mail Yoshitada_Sakai@tmc.toray.co.jp

Saito A, Kawanishi H, Yamashita AC, Mineshima M (eds): High-Performance Membrane Dialyzers.
Contrib Nephrol. Basel, Karger, 2011, vol 173, pp 148–155

Polyester Polymer Alloy as a High-Performance Membrane

Tadaaki Igoshi · Narumi Tomisawa · Yoshinori Hori · Yoichi Jinbo

Nikkiso Co. Ltd, Tokyo, Japan

Abstract

Polyester polymer alloy (PEPA) membrane is developed as a synthetic polymer membrane. It consists of two polymers – polyethersulfone (PES) and polyarylate (PAR). The pore size in membrane can be controlled by a blend ratio of PES and PAR. One unique characteristic is that PEPA membrane has three layers of a skin layer on the inner surface, a porous layer in the membrane, and a skin layer on the outer surface, respectively. The permeability of water and substances is controlled by the skin layer on the inner surface. PEPA membrane dialyzer can be adequately considered as a high-performance dialyzer. Furthermore, the skin layer on the outer surface can block endotoxin from the dialysis fluid side. PEPA membrane can therefore be used as an endotoxin-retentive filter. The other unique characteristic is that each amount of albumin loss or β_2-microglobulin removal can be controlled by an additive amount of polyvinylpyrrolidone. This means that the PEPA dialyzer can be clinically used to meet the conditions of the patient.

Synthetic polymer membranes are widely used as dialysis membranes for hemodialyzer therapy. Polyester polymer alloy (PEPA) membrane is one such synthetic polymer membrane and consists of two polymers – polyethersulfone (PES) and polyarylate (PAR). PEPA membrane utilizes a polymer blend technology and creates a multicomponent polymer with strong points of each polymer. PEPA can produce membrane without a hydrophilizing agent and the appropriate pore size can be controlled easily by a mixture ratio of these two polymers. The characteristic and clinical data of PEPA as a high-performance membrane for hemodialysis and related therapies are described.

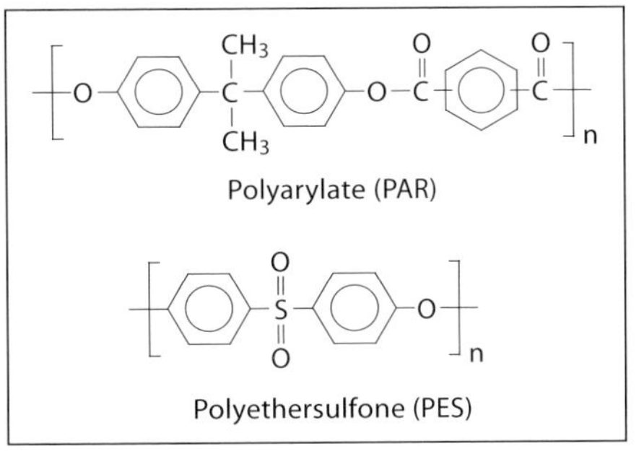

Fig. 1. Molecular structure of PEPA (PAR and PES).

Membrane Material and Types

Background on Development of PEPA Membrane

The main dialysis membrane was cellulose in the early 1970s, but many kinds of synthetic polymer membranes including polymethylmethacrylate or polyacrylonitrile had been developed. Because the synthetic polymer membranes had a high water permeability, filters with these membranes were used for hemofiltration therapy for the first time. Afterwards, dialysis machines equipped with an ultrafiltration controller became popular and synthetic membranes were also used for hemodialysis therapy. The new era had started. Moreover, there were so many reports that synthetic membranes were superior to cellulose membrane regarding biocompatibility. In 1985, β_2-microglobulin (β_2-MG) was identified as a causative substance of dialysis-related amyloidosis [1], and a dialysis membrane was strongly required to remove low-molecular protein. On the basis of this background, Nikkiso Co. established a technology to control the structure of dialysis membrane by blending of two kinds of polymer. In 1990, PEPA membrane was developed and met the performance requirements of the market.

PEPA Membrane

PEPA is polymer alloy blended with polymers and consists of PAR and PES. Alloying is one of the technologies to combine the good points of each polymer and to compensate the defects of each. PAR, one of the materials for PEPA, is an aromatic polyester polymer. In addition, it is a hydrophobic polymer with superior heat resistance, recovery performance, and mechanical properties. The other material, PES, is amorphous and a thermoplastic. As PAR, it is a hydrophobic polymer with superior heat resistance, chemical resistance and radiation such as γ- or X-ray resistance. The molecular structures of PAR and PES are shown in figure 1.

Hydrophilic PEPA Membrane

Hydrophilic PEPA membrane was developed in 2001 and is produced for hemodialysis therapy by improving blood compatibility to use polyvinylpyrrolidone

(PVP) as a hydrophilic agent. It becomes possible to control the adsorption of protein in blood by controlling hydrophilicity of the inner surface of hollow fibers with PEPA.

Manufacturing Process

Membrane Manufacturing Process

The manufacturing process of PEPA membrane can be outlined as follows. As a first step, two kinds of polymer, PAR and PES, are blended at a fixed ratio and dissolved with a solvent to produce a spinning dope. After the dope is uniformly mixed up and defoamed, it is discharged from a double-pipe spinning sleeve to a solidification solution in a bath. At the same time the core solution is discharged from the center of the double-pipe sleeve. The dope discharged from the double-pipe spinning sleeve is simultaneously contacted with both the solidification solution and core solution, and solidified from both the outside and inside of the hollow fiber by substituting solvent for water. The hollow fiber is produced in this process.

The solvent is completely removed in the washing process and PEPA membrane is finally completed after the drying process.

The main feature of PEPA membrane is that it needs no use of an additive such as pore formation agent in the manufacturing process. The general purpose of adding a pore formation agent is to form a suitable pore in the membrane by controlling the dissolution condition of polymer and by preventing rapid agglomeration of polymer in the spinning dope during solidification. For example, in the membrane formation of polysulfone, hydrosoluble polymer (such as polyethylene glycol, PVP) or alcohols are added to the spinning dope and a suitable pore is generally formed.

PEPA membrane can form a suitable pore without addition of a pore formation agent. The different solubility to the solvent between PAR and PES is strongly related with pore formation for PEPA membrane. Because solidification of PAR is faster than that of PES, it is supposed that coexisting PES prevents rapid agglomeration of PAR and in a succeeding agglomeration process of PES, coexisting PAR microgel prevents rapid agglomeration of PES. Therefore, if the blend ratio between PAR and PES is varied, each agglomeration speed continuously generated for PAR and PES can be controlled and this agglomeration speed is a factor for the decision of the membrane structure [2]. That is to say, variation of the blend ratio for two polymers has the possibility to produce a different performance of the PEPA membrane.

Dialyzer Manufacturing Process

The hollow fiber bundle for each membrane surface area is loaded into housing and both ends of the housing are filled with polyurethane, two liquids of

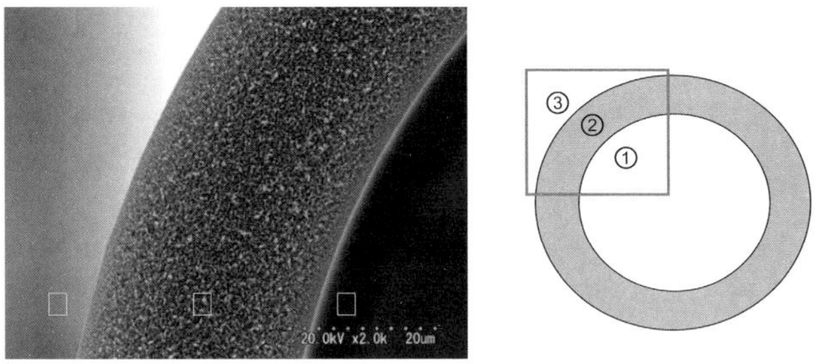

Unique three-layer structure:

① Blood side	Skin layer	Substance permeability
② Inside membrane	Porous layer	Mechanical strength
③ Dialysis fluid side	Skin layer	ET block

Fig. 2. Cross-sectional photograph of a hollow fiber showing the three layers.

hardening resin, as potting material. Next, both ends of the potting parts are cut with a cutting machine to open the closed hollow fiber. After capping of the housing, each module undergoes a leak test. At the same time, modules not passing the test are rejected. The passing modules are filled with purified water on both the blood side and dialysis fluid side. Finally, each module is sterilized with γ-rays as the final product.

Structure and Characteristic of Membranes

Membrane Structure

The structure of PEPA membrane is shown in figure 2. PEPA is an asymmetric structure membrane and has a three-layer structure, i.e. a skin layer on the inner surface, a support layer in the middle of range of thickness, and a skin layer on the outer surface. It is the inner skin layer with <1 μm thickness that determines the permeability from the blood side to the dialysis fluid side. The part between the two skin layers is a porous layer to maintain the membrane's strength and permeability.

The PEPA membrane has the characteristic to form a similar skin layer on the outer surface as the inner surface. This is a reason why PEPA has a different way to solidify compared with other synthetic polymers.

Elution of Hydrophilic Agent

As described above, production of PEPA membrane has the characteristic of not needing any additive such as pore formation agent. PVP is not eluted from the FL series because this series does not contain PVP. In view of the fact that

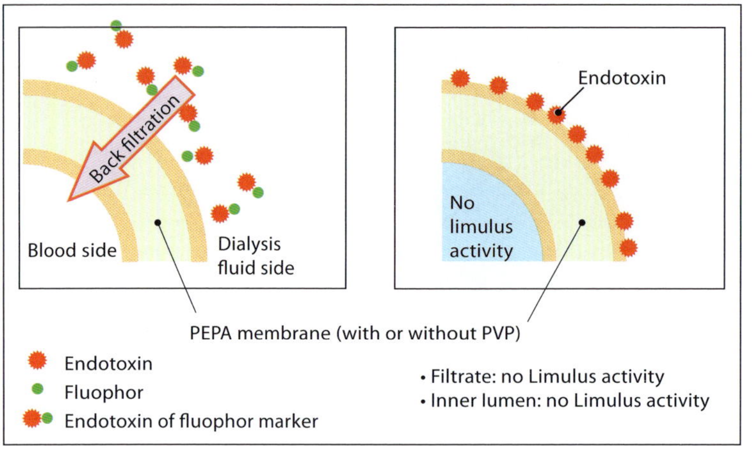

Fig. 3. Schematic diagram of the ET adsorption state.

the FD series has a minimum necessary amount of PVP added, it is checked whether very small amounts of PVP are eluted compared to other synthetic polymer membranes using PVP.

An elution test was done for the FD series using the following method: (a) draining and filling water from the blood side and dialysis fluid side of the dialyzer; (b) filling the dialysis fluid side with saline; (c) priming with 1 liter of saline in the blood side; (d) circulating 1 liter of saline for 4 h, and (e) measuring the PVP amount in saline using the Mueller method after completion of circulation. As a result, the elution amount was less than the measurement sensitivity for the FD series, including FDX and FDY.

Endotoxin Retentive Capability

It is reported that PEPA membrane has a superior endotoxin (ET) retentive capability. It is schematically outlined in figure 3 how ET is retentive on PEPA membrane [3]. A solution including ET labeled with fluorescent substance was passed through the PEPA membrane from the dialysis fluid side to the blood side, and the retentive ET was observed with a confocal scanning laser microscopy. ET was shown as the part generating green-colored fluorescence and it was clear that most of them were retentive on the skin layer of the outer surface. Therefore, this phenomenon does not seem to have any influence on blood. On the other hand, in other synthetic membranes without a skin layer on the outer surface, it is possible for ET to reach the skin layer on the inner surface and have a bad impact on blood. As described above, the PEPA membrane has a superior ET retentive ability and this ability is utilized for ET-retentive filters.

Table 1. Specification and performance of all types of PEPA dialyzer (in Japan)

Dialyzer		Technical data		Performance data				
					clearance (average Q_B = 200 ml/min)			
series	type	surface m^2	volume ml	UF factor ml/mm Hg/h	urea ml/min	creatinine ml/min	phosphate ml/min	vitamin B_{12} ml/min
FL	FLX-08GW	0.8	50	24	176	164	150	109
	FLX-10GW	1.0	60	28	181	171	167	127
	FLX-12GW	1.2	76	34	186	177	173	137
	FLX-15GW	1.5	92	39	193	184	180	150
	FLX-18GW	1.8	108	47	197	192	190	168
	FLX-21GW	2.1	135	50	198	194	193	174
FD	FDX-80GW	0.8	50	32	170	155	145	102
	FDX-100GW	1.0	58	40	180	168	155	116
	FDX-120GW	1.2	72	45	186	176	168	128
	FDX-150GW	1.5	91	50	190	183	177	142
	FDX-180GW	1.8	108	57	192	186	178	155
	FDX-210GW	2.1	126	63	193	187	181	159
	FDY-100GW	1.0	58	41	180	170	155	120
	FDY-120GW	1.2	72	46	186	176	168	134
	FDY-150GW	1.5	91	52	191	184	178	146
	FDY-180GW	1.8	108	59	193	186	181	156
	FDY-210GW	2.1	126	63	194	187	183	161
	FDY-250GW	2.5	146	67	198	196	188	168
	FDY-15GW	1.5	91	51	191	181	176	147
	FDY-18GW	1.8	108	59	192	186	180	155
	FDY-21GW	2.1	126	63	194	189	183	162

Membrane: polyester-polymer alloy; membrane diameter: 210 μm; wall thickness 30 μm; sterilization: gamma sterilization.

Specification and Performance for Dialyzers

Specification

All dialyzers are the water-filling type and sterilized with γ-rays. Each specification of the FL series with PEPA membrane and the FD series with hydrophilic PEPA membrane is listed in table 1, respectively.

Performance

The performance of FLX, FDX, and FDY is also shown in table 1. All types have high a removal performance of low-molecular substances and high permeability of water. They also have high removal permeability for β_2-MG (MW 11,800), the causative substance of dialysis-related amyloidosis. Moreover, the hydrophilic PEPA dialyzer has been improved, such as downsized housing and a smoothed cutting surface of polyurethane [4]. The FD series, hydrophilic PEPA dialyzer, has two different types of water permeability: FDX and FDY. The various PEPA and hydrophilic PEPA dialyzer models are listed in table 1.

Clinical Evaluation

Removal Performance

Each type of PEPA dialyzer has sufficient performance for low-molecular-weight substances [5]. There seems to be a significant difference between PEPA and other synthetic membrane dialyzers. On the other hand, β_2-MG of one of the low-molecular-weight proteins was removed enough, e.g. (i) removal rate for FLX-150GW 58.0 ± 6.5% [6] and FDY-150GW 68.6 ± 4.1% [7] in hemodialysis (HD) treatment, and (ii) FDY-150GW 77.4 ± 4.1% [7] in hemodiafiltration (HDF) treatment.

Albumin Loss

The amount of albumin loss was <1 g/session in a case of HD treatment with FDX-150GW [6]. This means that the FDX dialyzer is suitable in patients where there is a need to remove a certain amount of β_2-MG but to minimize albumin loss. In the case of a 50-liter pre-dilution HDF treatment with FDY-150GW, the amount of albumin loss was 3.2 ± 0.7 g/session [7]. It is supposed that this larger loss of albumin stimulates new albumin formation. Therefore, the FDY dialyzer (100 series) seems to be suitable for patients with the ability to metabolize in order to cover the amount of albumin loss. As this dialyzer is used as a filter for massive substitution of pre-dilution HDF, it is possible to improve the symptoms of patients with a dialysis syndrome.

Biocompatibility

PEPA membrane has an excellent ET trap from the membrane construction. In clinical use, a patient's fever ceased after switching from a PS dialyzer to a PEPA membrane (FLX dialyzer) [8]. The reason is supposed that the PEPA membrane prevented ET coming into contact with blood from dialysis fluid. Regarding complement activation, plasma levels of C3a and C5a were low during hemodialysis [5]. The FLX dialyzer was used for this clinical evaluation and it showed that PEPA membrane without PVP hardly activated complements. Besides these data it was reported that there was a relationship between additive amounts of PVP and concentration of C3a, and a small additional amount of PVP could control activation of complements [9]. From another viewpoint, an example was given that plasma free light chain was removed in a patient with primary amyloidosis by HDF treatment with PEPA (FLX dialyzer) [10]. Although only a few cases have been reported, a FLX dialyzer could be used as a therapy in those with primary amyloidosis.

References

1 Gejyo F, Yamada T, Odani S, Nakagawa Y, Arakawa M, Kunitomo T, Kataoka H, Suzuki M, Hirasawa Y, Shirahama T, Cohen AS, Schmid K: A new form of amyloid protein associated with chronic hemodialysis was identified as β_2-microglobulin. Biochem Biophys Res Commun 1985;129:701–706.

2 Shimizu M, Kanamori T, Sakai K, Igoshi T, Yoshida M: New polymer alloy dialysis membranes with varying permeabilities and sievings. Am Soc Artif Intern Organs 1992;38:784–787.

3 Hayama M, Miyasaka T, Mochizuki S, Asahara H, Yamamoto K, Kohori F, Tsujioka K, Sakai K: Optimum dialysis membrane for endotoxin blocking. J Membr Sci 2003;219:15–25.

4 Nakamura T, Oka I, Ehara S, Hukushima A, Isezaki R, Aoki S, Kihara N, Nakata M, Okazaki T, Matsufuji A, Toyada K, Tokuyama M: Performance evaluation of FDY-150GW (in Japanese). Jin To Toseki 2004;57:S61–S65.

5 Stein J, Guenther K, Sperschneider H, Carlsohn H, Hueller M, Schubert K, Schaller R: Clinical evaluation of a new dialyzer, FLX-12GW, with a polyester-polymer alloy membrane. Artif Organs 1993;17:339–345.

6 Goto H, Hasegawa F, Megumi R, Megumi I, Nakao M, Sekiya M: Performance evaluation FDX-150GW with modified hydrophilic PEPA membrane (in Japanese). Jin To Toseki 2004;57:S56–S60.

7 Saito T, Yamauchi F, Tsukahara T, Kanazawa Y, Hattori K, Asahi D, Sakurai K, Yamashita A: Performance evaluation of modified FDX-150GW in HD and pre-dilution online HDF (in Japanese). Jin To Toseki 2006;61S97–S102.

8 Murata T, Nakamura T, Yoshitake K, Enomoto M, Michinaga I, Yoshizawa S, Ogawara S, Naito S: An example of conventional hemodialysis patient affected by aluminum encephalopathy disappearing fever after HDF treatment with FLX dialyzer (in Japanese). Proc Kyushu Soc HDF Therapy, 1995, vol 1, pp 7–9.

9 Yamashita A, Tomisawa N, Takezawa A, Sakurai K, Sakai T: Blood compatibility and filtration characteristics of a newly developed polyester polymer alloy membrane. Hemodial Int 2004;8:368–371.

10 Machiguchi T, Tamura T, Yoshida H: Efficacy of haemodiafiltration treatment with PEPA dialysis membranes in plasma free light chain removal in a patient with primary amyloidosis. Nephrol Dial Transplant 2002,17:1689–1691.

Tadaaki Igoshi
Nikkiso Co. Ltd, 43-2, Ebisu 3-Chome
Shibuya-ku, Tokyo 150-8677 (Japan)
Tel. +81 3 3443 3756
E-Mail T.Igoshi@nikkiso.co.jp

Saito A, Kawanishi H, Yamashita AC, Mineshima M (eds): High-Performance Membrane Dialyzers.
Contrib Nephrol. Basel, Karger, 2011, vol 173, pp 156–163

Cellulose Triacetate as a High-Performance Membrane

Takashi Sunohara · Toshiaki Masuda

Nipro Corporation, Dialysis-Related Products, Osaka, Japan

Abstract

The cellulose triacetate membrane is one of the typical high-performance membranes. Cellulose triacetate is a plastic material manufactured from cellulose. The hydroxyl group of cellulose is chemically substituted for the carboxyl group. Therefore, its characteristics are quite different from cellulose. The cellulose triacetate membrane has a homogeneous membrane structure. It can be produced with a wide range of permeability, from low-flux performance to super high-flux performance. Because the thickness of the membrane is thin, and flow distribution of the dialysate (due to the moiré structure) is uniform, this enables the development of a dialyzer with high diffusive efficiency. Recently, this new product, improved through a sieving process, produced a uniform pore size distribution. As for the dialyzer, through sterilization by γ-rays with the absence of oxygen, now enables long-term safety of the product. Several clinical improvements have been reported, such as high antithrombus, the improvement of lipid metabolism and the reduction of biomarkers. Thus, continuous membrane development is desired, made of safe and stable cellulose triacetate material.

The cellulose triacetate membrane was clinically used as a dialysis membrane made of cellulose triacetate in the 1980s. It has material characteristics and surface characteristics quite different from the regenerated cellulose. Therefore, clinical utility was widely evaluated. Its reported stability and biocompatibilities are different from the dialysis membranes that are made of other synthetic polymers. It has a lot of features including a high solute permeability that can remove the β_2-microglobulin by diffusion [1] and uniform dialysate flow, etc. Recently, a new cellulose triacetate membrane that showed a higher removal property was developed.

Material Features

The cellulose triacetate is produced as a result of a chemical reaction between the natural polymer cellulose and acetic acid. This is one kind of cellulose-based plastic [2], industrialized in 1922. Cellulose triacetate is used for many manufactured products, such as the protective film of liquid crystal panels. In application as a membrane, its use is not limited to dialysis, but it can also used as a reverse osmotic membrane, etc. Triacetate and diacetate are used as membrane material. The substitution degree of the hydroxyl groups in cellulose is almost 3 for triacetate and almost 2.5 for diacetate. The higher the substitution degree, the more hydrophilic it becomes. Thus, diacetate is an excellent industrial material for this process. It is a material that does not generate harmful gases such as NOx and SOx during incineration because the cellulose acetate is only composed by carbon, oxygen, and hydrogen.

Spinning Method of Triacetate Hollow-Fiber Membrane

There are two methods for spinning the membrane of the cellulose triacetate hollow-fiber membrane [3, 4]; the melt spinning method and the wet spinning method. In the melt spinning method the cellulose acetate is heated to 240–280°C with the plasticizer. Next, after it melts, it is exhaled from the double circular tube nozzle. It is manufactured through the process of cooling, washing in clear water, resulting in re-plasticity and dryness. The phase separation happens when the melting polymer, due to the exhaled high temperature, is cooled by the nozzle. Fine pores are formed within the membrane at this time. On the other hand, in the wet spinning method, the membrane is mixed and dissolved with the solvent of the cellulose acetate. It is similarly exhaled from the double circular tube nozzle, and coagulates. At this time, coagulation occurs due to the removal of the solvent in the phase separation, and fine pores are formed in membrane. In both spinning methods, the solvent is washed out continuously. Before the drying process, the membrane is passed through a glycerin bath to maintain fine pore size, and to keep it hydrophilic, the glycerin fills in the pores. As for the glycerin in the membrane, the solubility into water is very high. Before it is used, the dialyzer is primed with saline, and the glycerin is completely removed. As for spinning of the hollow-fiber membrane, diacetate was previously industrialized. Melting points are lower than triacetate, and the dissolubility of diacetate is higher. Later, high productivity was established for triacetate. It is easy to control pore size of the hollow-fiber membrane of cellulose triacetate in system cellulose thermoplastic plastic. Therefore, different performances of membranes are developed by changing the membrane manufacturing process.

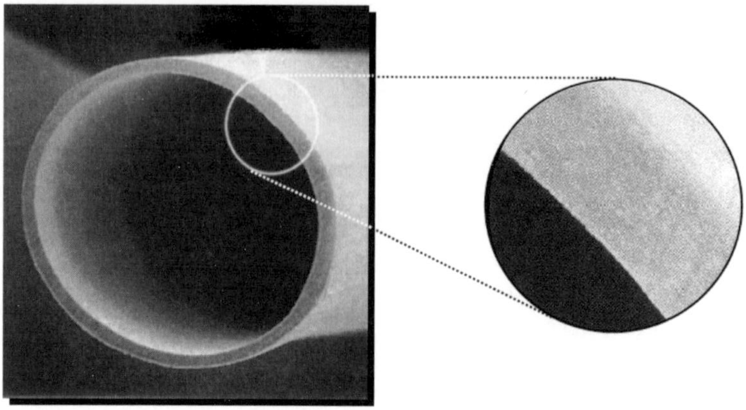

Fig. 1. Cross-sectional structure of cellulose triacetate membrane.

Features of Cellulose Triacetate Membrane Dialyzers

Membrane Structure and Solute Permeability Characteristic

The cellulose triacetate membrane is the thinnest dialysis membrane at 15 μm on the market. There is no water absorption property like cellulose because there are few highly hydrophilic hydroxyl groups. There are few dimensional changes in the dry and wet states.

The cross-sectional structure of the membrane is uniform. Pore size of the inside and outside of the hollow fiber is almost the same. Pore size on the outer surface of the membrane is relatively smaller than a general asymmetric membrane. Therefore, backfiltration of endotoxin and the bacillus origin material that exists in the dialysate does not occur easily. Oppositely, the pore size of the inner surface of membrane is relatively bigger than that of an asymmetric structural membrane. After blood comes into contact with the membrane's inner side, a uniform protein layer is formed. It has been reported that the protein layer is uniform as albumin monolayer is formed. High demarcation characteristics are shown because pore size becomes appropriate for that protein layer.

The range of cellulose triacetate membrane available at present varies from low flux to the super high flux. Clearance myoglobin, whose molecular weight is 17,000, greatly changes according to the control of each average pore radius and the rate of pore density. β_2-Microglobulin clearance ranges from about 10 ml/min to about 70 ml/min when the membrane surface area of the dialyzer is 1.5 m^2. To achieve the high clearance of β_2-microglobulin, while keeping the albumin leakage small to moderate, as is common in recent years, a higher sieving characteristic is needed. Therefore, a new spinning technology that extremely improves the separation characteristics of the triacetate membrane was developed. It became possible to arrange pore size uniformly by improving the spinning technology contrary to previous methods (fig. 1; table 1).

Table 1. Technical data of cellulose triacetate membrane dialyzers

Japanese brand/ international brand	Japanese classification	Pore radius Å	Porosity %	Urea clearance ml/min	Myoglobin clearance ml/min
FB-UHβ/no brand	class V	77	82	199	96
FB-FH/Sureflux-FH	class IV	78	84	198	78
FB-Uβ/Sureflux-UX	class IV	72	78	198	67
FB-UH/Sureflux-UH	class III	76	80	198	69
FB-F/no brand	class III	75	73	198	62
FB-U	class III	70	70	196	39
FB-P/no brand	class III	68	69	193	32
FB-E/Sureflux-E	class II	63	67	191	25
FB-G/Sureflux-G	class II	60	65	191	20
FB-EG/Sureflux-L	class I	58	63	191	7

Uniform Dialysate Flow Distribution by the Moiré Structure

It is necessary to optimize the flow of blood and the dialysate to enhance the solute removal characteristics of the dialysis membrane to its maximum and to improve the performance of the dialyzer. The dialysate flows on the outside of the hollow-fiber membrane in a dialyzer. A slight meander is given to the cellulose acetate membrane. It flows uniformly in the dialysate between the outside of the hollow-fiber membrane. This slight meander sees externals of the hollow-fiber membrane and the pattern that looks like moiré fringes. This is called a moiré structure. Figure 2 is the observation resulting from using helical X-rays CT [5]. As for the dialyzer of the moiré structure, the effect that the dialysate flows uniformly was confirmed.

Biocompatibility

In cellulose triacetate, the hydroxyl groups that existed in the chemical structure of cellulose are substituted by the acetyl group during the synthesis process of the raw material. The hydroxyl groups are responsible for the activation of complement during dialysis. The activation of complement is decreased in the cellulose triacetate membrane. Changes of the activity of complement are negligible and the white blood cell count under the dialysis is reported to be few, as well [6, 7]. Moreover, data have been reported showing few changes in the granulocyte elastase and the platelet numbers. Moreover, the PCOOH elevation dialyzed with triacetate membrane is reported to be lower than that of cellulose membrane [8]. It causes few oxidant stresses for the triacetate membrane.

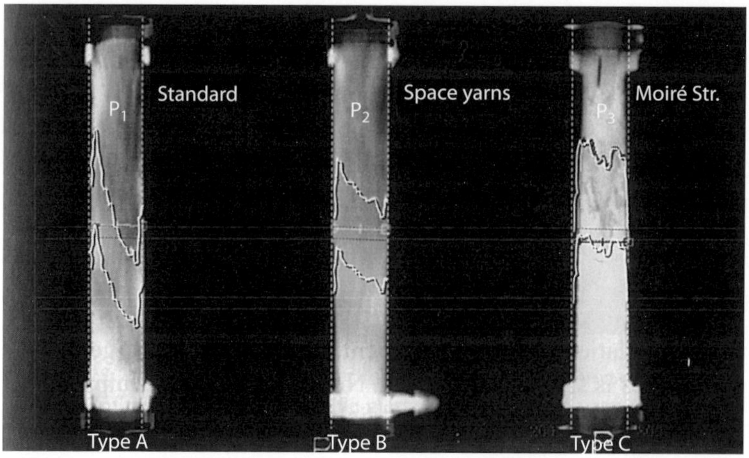

Fig. 2. Flow rate distribution of dialysate in three types of dialyzer [from ref. 5]: type A: standard straight hollow-fiber dialyzer; type B: straight hollow fiber with space yarns dialyzer, and type C: moiré structure hollow-fiber dialyzer.

Adsorption Characteristics

The electrical charge of a dialysis membrane has an influence on adsorption characteristics during clinical use of the dialyzer. As for the triacetate membrane whose electrical charge is low, the adsorption of the protein or the medicine is reported to be minimal [9]. Moreover, when the electrical charge of a membrane is low, a high phosphorus clearance is reported. Besides this, there are reports of improvement of the disorder lipid metabolism, described later, about the adsorption of the serum lipid [10].

Sterilization [11]

The cellulose triacetate membrane can be sterilized by gamma sterilization, steam sterilization under pressure, and EOG sterilization.

When a polymer is exposed to γ-rays, free radicals are formed through ionization and excitation of the polymer. Free radical dissipation degrades the polymer. We have found that the reaction can be restrained under conditions where oxygen is not present. Cellulose triacetate dialyzers have been exposure to γ-rays after packing in gas-impermeable bags (aluminum-laminated plastic film) together with an oxygen absorber. No deterioration in strength or charge was detected in the extraction of materials after 5 years in storage. Biological tests on the materials and dialyzers all gave acceptable results and safety could be maintained for at least 5 years. The dose of γ-rays for sterilization is proportional to the presumed number of microorganisms on the dialyzers. To achieve more stable sterilization, the number of microorganisms must be minimized. By keeping the production facility clean it is possible to produce dialyzers with

Table 2. Clinical reports of biomarker reduction

Study	Evaluated dialyzer	Biomarkers	Removal result
Van Tellingen [17]	FB-150F	homocysteine	33% reduction
De Vriese [18]	FB-150FH	homocysteine	15% reduction
De Smet [19]	Sureflux-150FH	indoxyl sulfate	32.5% reduction
		AGEs	55.8% reduction

a very low number of microorganisms throughout the year. On this basis, it is concluded that the low sterilization dose should achieve an adequate level of sterility (10^{-6}).

The dialyzer of the gamma sterilization of a dry type is a product that resists a strong impact because it is light, and safe, without the risk of leakage, such as hollow fibers freezing in the regions where it is cold.

Characteristics of Clinical Application

Excellent Antithrombus

As for the cellulose triacetate membrane dialyzer, it is reported it has a high antithrombus performance. After being used for clinical dialysis, there is little residual blood loss [12]. Especially the decrease in platelet counts is reported to be negligible with the triacetate membrane, while those using polysulfone membrane dialyzers decreased [13–15]. As for the triacetate membrane, it is reported that the cohesion of the platelet is not generated, because the change in the platelet surface structure is not caused easily in relation to this event [16].

Improvement of Lipid Metabolism

As for the cellulose triacetate membrane, the balance of hydrophilic and hydrophobic is properly controlled. Therefore, APO-CIII is removed by adsorption on triacetate membrane. Triglycerides decreased when the triacetate membrane was used for long periods, and data showing that the HDL cholesterol increases have been reported [10].

Improvement of Biomarkers

As for the cellulose triacetate membrane, there have been reports of two or more life prolongments of the dialyzed patient and the improvement of biomarker data. Especially, data that is much better than other membrane materials is reported and reports of the decrease of homocysteine, sometimes related to cardiovascular complications mental illnesses (table 2).

Conclusion

The cellulose triacetate membrane is an excellent material in terms of biocompatibility. It is hoped there will be a continuous development of new membranes corresponding to clinical demands in the future, with potential characteristics where removal properties can be widely controlled.

References

1 Naitoh A, Tatsuguchi T, Okada M, Ohmura T, Sakai K: Removal of β_2-microglobulin by diffusion alone is feasible using highly permeable dialysis membranes. Trans Am Soc Artif Intern Organs 1988;34:630–634.

2 Kroschwitz JT: Cellulose Esters. Organic Encyclopedia of Polymer Science and Engineering. New York, Wiley-Interscience, 1987, vol 3, p 166.

3 Masuda T, Fukui K: Cellulose triacetate as membrane material; in Cellulose Triacetate. Milan, Wichting Editore, 1994, pp 9–20.

4 Masuda T: Modified cellulose triacetate membranes. Hemodialysis technology. Contrib Nephrol. Basel, Karger, 2002, vol 137, pp 106–110.

5 Ronco C, Brendolan A, Dell'Aquila R, Tasinazzo L, Bettini MC, Greca GL: Impact of diffusion coefficients and membrane structure on phosphate clearance in hemodialysis; in Cellulose Triacetate. Milan, Wichtig Editore, 1994, pp 75–85.

6 Jacques C, Sylvie L, Christine R, Philippe R: New insights in dialysis membrane biocompatibility: relevance of adsorption properties and heparin binding. Nephrol Dial Transplant 2003;18:253–257.

7 Hoenich NA, Woffindin C, Mathews JN, Vinken J: Biocompatibility of membranes used in the treatment of renal failure. Biomaterials 1995;16:587–592.

8 Sanaka T, Higuchi C, Shinobe T, Nishimura H, Omata M, Nihei H, Sugino N: Lipid peroxidation as an indicator of biocompatibility in haemodialysis. Nephrol Dial Transplant 1995;10(suppl 3):34–38.

9 Renaux JL, Thomas M, Crost T, Loughraieb N, Vantard G: Activation of the kallikrein-kinin system in hemodialysis: role of membrane electoronegativity, blood dilution, and pH. Kidney Int 1999;55:1097–1103.

10 Otsubo Y, Tabe T, Takenouchi K, Toyama M, Uruta Y, Yasumoto Y, Uchida Y, Arima T: Lipid metabolism in dialyzed patients treated with CTA membrane; in Cellulose Triacetate. Milan Wichting, 1994, pp 161–170.

11 Masuda T, Fukui K: Gamma sterilization of cellulose triacetate dialyzers; in Cellulose Triacetate. Milan, Wichting Editore, 1994, pp 35–44.

12 Kalocheretis P, Vlamis L, Belesi C, Makriniotou I, Zerbala S, Savidou E, Zorbas S, Arvanitis N, Iatrou C: Residual blood loss in single use dialyzers: effect of different membranes and flux. Int J Artif Organs 2006;29:286–292.

13 Shuangxin L, Wei S, Xinling L, Yong S, Yongzhen L, Bin Z, Zhiming Y, Lixia X, Yunfeng X, Chaoshen H, Jianchao M, Yiming T, Hen Y, Hui L: Cellulose triacetate dialyzer reduces platelet loss during continuous veno-venous hemofiltration. Blood Purif 2010;29:375–382.

14 Stefoni S, De Sanctis LB, Cianciolo G, Coli L, Buscaroli A, Feliciangeli G, Borgnino LC, Bonetti M, Gregorini MC, DeGiovanni P, Buttazzi R: Effect of different dialysis on platelet function. A mean for biocompatibility evaluation; in Cellulose Triacetate. Milan, Wichting Editore, 1994, pp 171–184.

15 De Sanctis LB, Stefoni S, Cianciolo G, Coli L, Buscaroli A, Feliciangeli G, Borgnino LC, Bonetti M, Gregorini MC, Giovanni PD, Buttazzi R: Effect of different dialysis membranes on platelet function. A tool for biocompatibility evaluation. Int J Artif Organs 1996;19:404–410.

16 Kuragano T, Kuno T, Takahashi Y, Yamamoto C, Nagura Y, Takahashi S, Kanmatsuse K: Comparison of the effects of cellulose triacetate and polysulfone membrane on GPIIb/IIIa and platelet activation. Blood Purif 2003;21:176–182.
17 Van Tellingen A, Grooteman MP, Bartels PC, van Limbeek J, van Guldener C, Wee PM, Nubé MJ: Long-term reduction in plasma homocysteine levels by super-flux dialyzers in hemodialysis patients. Kidney Int 2001;59:342 –347.
18 De Vriese AS, Langlois M, Bernard D, Geerolf I, Stevens L, Boelaert JR, Schurgers M, Matthys E: Effect of dialyser membrane pore size on plasma homocysteine levels in haemodialysis patients. Nephrol Dial Transplant 2003;18:2596–2600.
19 De Smet R, Dhondt A, Eloot S, Galli F, Waterloos MA, Vanholder R: Effect of the super-flux cellulose triacetate dialyser membrane on the removal of non-protein-bound and protein-bound uraemic solutes. Nephrol Dial Transplant 2007;22:2006–2012.

Takashi Sunohara
Nipro Corporation, Dialysis-Related Products
3-3-13, Toyosaki, Kita-ku, Osaka 531-0072 (Japan)
Tel. +81 6 6373 0092
E-Mail sunohara-takashi@nipro.co.jp

Saito A, Kawanishi H, Yamashita AC, Mineshima M (eds): High-Performance Membrane Dialyzers.
Contrib Nephrol. Basel, Karger, 2011, vol 173, pp 164–171

Ethylene Vinyl Alcohol Co-Polymer as a High-Performance Membrane: An EVOH Membrane with Excellent Biocompatibility

Akiyoshi Nakano

EV Plant, Blood Purification Business Unit, Asahi Kasei Kuraray Medical Co. Ltd, Nobeoka, Miyazaki, Japan

Abstract

Over the last few years, with an increase in the number of patients receiving long-term dialysis and elderly patients on dialysis, the frequency of cardiovascular complications and complications associated with long-term dialysis have increased sharply. As a result, dialysis treatment must be capable of reducing oxidative stress and mitigating the inflammatory response. The ethylene vinyl alcohol (EVOH) co-polymer is a hydrophilic and uncharged synthetic polymer blend. EVOH membranes have a smooth surface and retain structural water, so they adsorb few plasma proteins. Dialysis using an EVOH membrane results in minimal platelet activation and little generation of reactive oxygen species by activated neutrophils. Consequently, patients have good peripheral circulation. As a result, fluid containing uremic toxins moves readily from the intracellular compartment to the intravascular compartment through the interstitial space. In addition, these membranes cause minimal activation of coagulation during dialysis; therefore, genes encoding monocyte chemoattractant protein-1 and inflammatory cytokines (e.g. IL-6) are expressed at low levels. Thus, treatment involving an EVOH membrane can be expected to help alleviate cardiovascular complications and complications of dialysis.

The resin used to make ethylene vinyl alcohol (EVOH) co-polymer hollow fibers is a random co-polymer of ethylene and vinyl alcohol. Ethylene and vinyl acetate are co-polymerized by solution polymerization, and the co-polymer obtained is saponified using an alkali catalyst to manufacture the resin (fig. 1). The characteristics of the EVOH membrane are as follows: (1) the membrane is hydrophilic, so it need not contain hydrophilic substances like polyvinylpyrrolidone

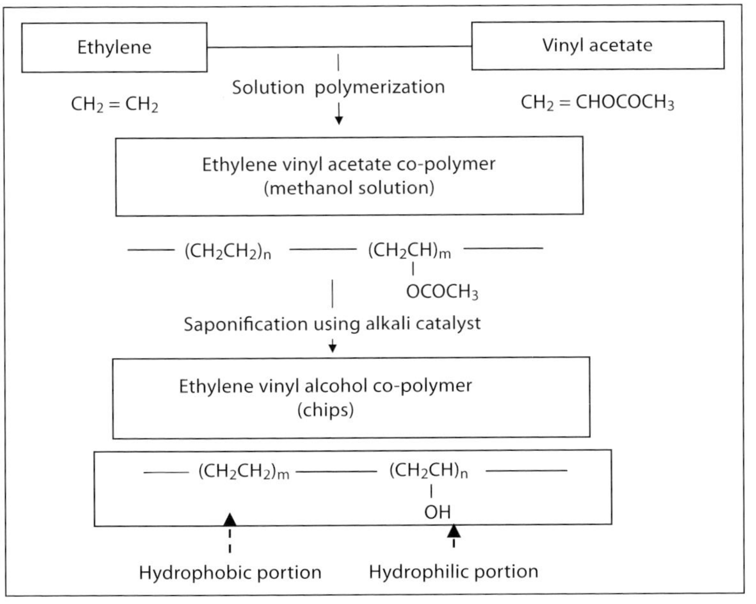

Fig. 1. EVOH resin manufacturing process.

Table 1. Specifications of three EVOH dialysis membranes

Membrane specifications	D	m	C
Inner diameter, μm		175	
Thickness, μm		25	
UFR, ml/mm Hg/h/m^2	5.8	7.7	8.7
β_2-MG SC	0.49	0.65	0.65
Albumin SC	0.02	0.03	0.04
Product name	Hollow fiber dialyzer KF- 201		

(PVP); (2) the membrane is uncharged, and (3) when it contains water, the membrane surface is smooth and pliable and retains structural water. There are three versions of EVOH dialysis membranes: D, m, and C (table 1).

In vitro Assessment of EVOH Membranes

Membrane Structure, Performance, and Biocompatibility

SEM images of an EVOH membrane are shown in figure 2. The EVOH membrane has a homogeneous structure resulting in less risk of backfiltration

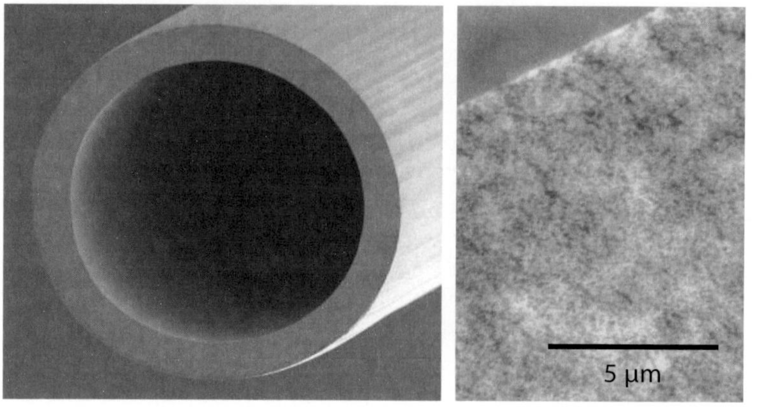

Fig. 2. SEM images of the EVOH membrane.

compared to an asymmetric membrane. In addition, the EVOH membrane has relatively large pores, which provide the membrane with extensive removal properties akin to those of a functioning kidney and allow removal of solutes with middle- and large-sized molecules.

Atomic force microscopy was performed to assess the roughness of the inner surface (depth of projections and depressions) of an EVOH membrane, a cellulose diacetate (CDA) membrane, and a polysulfone (PS) membrane in water, and the results of atomic force microscopy indicated that the EVOH membrane had the smoothest inner surface. In addition, assessment of the mobility of polymer chains using pulsed ^{13}C-NMR indicated that the EVOH membrane had greater interaction with water molecules than did membranes of other materials, and the EVOH membrane had highly mobile molecular chains. An EVOH membrane retains structural water on the membrane surface, so it adsorbs few plasma proteins and interacts weakly with the cell components in blood. Thus, this membrane has exceptional blood compatibility [1, 2].

Typically, when blood contacts a dialysis membrane, the body's lines of defense react: (1) plasma proteins adsorb to the membrane surface; (2) the adsorbed proteins are denatured, and then (3) the cellular components of blood are activated and adhere to the membrane. An EVOH membrane inhibits the adsorption of plasma proteins, thereby inhibiting the body's reaction to the membrane [3–8].

Reaction of Blood Cells upon Contact with a Dialysis Membrane

Since dialysis membranes are repeatedly in contact blood over time, they should ideally have little effect on the body. The effects of an EVOH membrane on blood have been assessed in vitro, and this membrane has been reported to have little effect on platelets and the coagulation system [9, 10].

Platelets are activated when blood comes into contact with a dialysis membrane. Tsuji et al. [3] used cell ELISA to measure P-selectin that is expressed on platelets and found a correlation between platelet adhesion and induction of P-selectin expression. The platelet adhesion and P-selectin expression associated with an EVOH membrane were lower than those associated with a PS membrane or polymethylmethacrylate (PMMA) membrane.

When neutrophils isolated from peripheral blood were labeled with a hydrogen peroxide (H_2O_2)-sensitive fluorescent dye (dichlorodihydrofluorescein diacetate, DCFH-DA) and brought into contact with a PS or PMMA membrane in the presence of platelets, they were found to produce reactive oxygen species (ROS) (fluorescence). In contrast, ROS were not induced when neutrophils came into contact with the EVOH membrane.

In vivo Assessment of EVOH Membranes

Removal Performance

EVOH membranes are biocompatible, and they show specific solute-removal properties and the capacity to mediate material transfer within the patient's body. In a crossover study of 12 patients, Oikawa et al. [7] compared the solute-removal properties of an EVOH membrane with those of a reformed cellulose (RC) membrane. Their assessment indicated that the urea clearance (K) and Kt/V associated with the EVOH membrane were significantly lower than those with the RC membrane. Conversely, the level of clearance as advocated by Barth [11] was higher and the hematocrit level was significantly lower when the EVOH membrane was used. This may be because solute transfer from the interior to the exterior of cells (plasma refilling) in dialysis treatment with the EVOH membrane was higher than that with the RC membrane. Thus, the EVOH membrane may have served to increase clearance despite the low K and Kt/V values.

Clinical Effectiveness

Maintenance of Peripheral Circulation

During dialysis, the interaction between blood and the dialysis membrane and the interaction between blood cells and the membrane alters the properties of blood and affects vascular endothelial cells and peripheral circulation. In a crossover study of 11 patients on dialysis, Sato et al. [6] used an EVOH membrane, a vitamin E-bonded cellulose (VE-C) membrane, and a PS membrane, and they measured transcutaneous oxygen ($TcPO_2$) at the dorsum of the foot and the fluidity of blood during dialysis. They found that use of the EVOH membrane moderated the decline in $TcPO_2$ during initial dialysis, in comparison with the decline associated with the use of the PS membrane and VE-C membrane. They

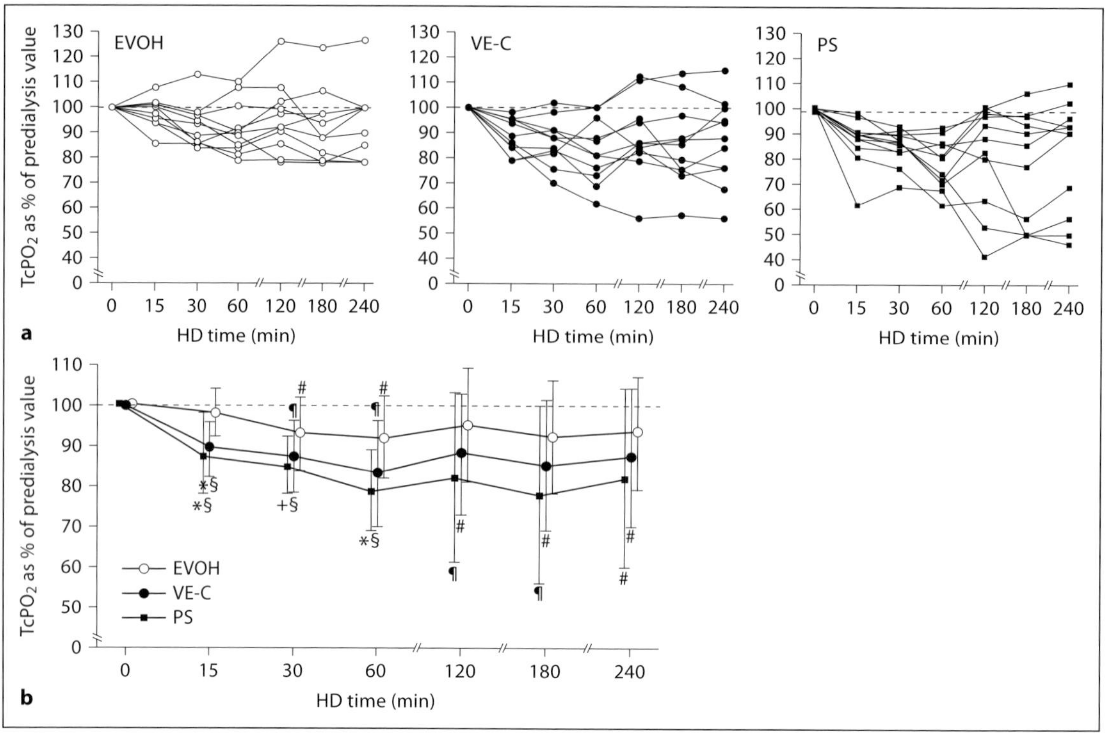

Fig. 3. **a** Changes in $TcPO_2$ during hemodialysis using EVOH, VE-C and PS membranes. **b** Results are percentages expressed as mean ± SD values. § $p < 0.005$, ¶ $p < 0.01$, $^{\#}$ $p < 0.05$ vs. predialysis (0 min) values for each membrane, * $p < 0.01$, $^{+}$ $p < 0.05$ vs. EVOH [from 6].

also indicated that the EVOH membrane was less apt to produce disturbances in peripheral circulation (fig. 3). Furthermore, diminished blood fluidity was not noted with the EVOH membrane. This is presumably because the EVOH membrane had minimal interaction with blood cells during dialysis.

Attention has recently focused on the association between peripheral circulation and the dynamics of solute and water removal from the patient. Specifically, the maintenance of peripheral circulation during dialysis should lead to the removal of solute from throughout the patient's body and relieve hypotension during dialysis.

Aggregates of Different Types of Cells and ROS Production during Dialysis

Contact between a dialysis membrane and blood is linked to biological processes such as the activation of blood cells, the formation of platelet-leukocyte (neutrophils or mononuclear cells) aggregates and platelet-erythrocyte aggregates, inflammation, congestion, and atherogenesis. In particular, neutrophils activated by interaction with platelets cause enhanced production of ROS,

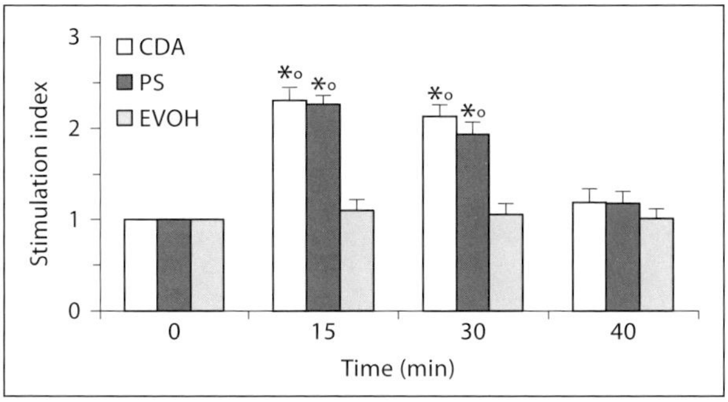

Fig. 4. ROS (hydrogen peroxide) production by the neutrophil population during hemodialysis with CDA, PS, and EVOH membranes. Production of hydrogen peroxide is expressed as a stimulation index (x-fold increase over production at start of dialysis). * $p < 0.05$ vs. predialysis. ° Significantly different from EVOH. [modified figure from 5].

which are believed to be associated with the complications of dialysis. Bonomini et al. [4, 5] performed whole-blood flow cytometry using various dialyzers to compare the platelet-leukocyte aggregation and platelet and leukocyte activation associated with each dialyzer. They measured P-selectin (CD62P), a marker of platelet activation, and deemed that leukocytes expressing CD62P on their surface (neutrophils or mononuclear cells) were platelet-leukocyte aggregates. They found that platelets activated by dialysis adhered to neutrophils and that these neutrophils were actually responsible for producing ROS. In addition, these steps differ depending on the dialysis membrane. Dialysis with an EVOH membrane significantly reduced platelet activation, platelet-neutrophil aggregates, and ROS production (fig. 4) in comparison to dialysis with a CDA membrane or a PS membrane.

Inflammatory Responses Caused by Activation of the Coagulation System

When the coagulation system is activated during dialysis, activated coagulation factor X (FXa) is released locally. FXa binds to specific receptors, such as effector protease receptor 1 (EPR-1) and protease-activated receptors (PARs), and activates peripheral blood mononuclear cells (PBMCs). Activation of PBMCs causes the release of a series of proinflammatory chemicals like cytokines, ROS, nitric oxide (NO), and monocyte chemoattractant protein-1 (MCP-1). In a crossover study of 10 patients undergoing dialysis with a cellulose acetate (CA) membrane or an EVOH membrane, Pertosa et al. [8] assessed the expression of genes associated with coagulation factor-specific receptors, signal transduction, and cytokines in PBMCs. They examined the inflammatory response in relation to a potential clotting reaction during dialysis. Along with a marked increase in the levels of stress-responsive kinases (e.g. JNK and ERK) and cytoplasm tyrosine kinase (Src), amplified expression of EPR-1, PAR-2, and PAR-4 mRNA was noted with the CA membrane, but little, if any, expression was detected with the EVOH membrane. In addition, amplified expression of CC chemokine receptor-2 (CCR2), MCP-1, and IL-6 mRNA was noted during use of the CA membrane, but minimal expression of these molecules was noted during use of the EVOH membrane. In other research, in vitro assessment revealed that the expression of CCR2B was induced by FXa.

Conclusion

Numerous researchers have studied the biocompatibility of dialysis membranes using various parameters, but there are no uniform criteria for judging biocompatibility. Since dialysis membrane biocompatibility is reportedly associated with vascular disorders, cardiovascular disease, and the prognosis of patients on dialysis [12], reducing the oxidative stress generated and the inflammatory response produced during dialysis is crucial.

Because of the material's specific biocompatibility, dialysis with an EVOH membrane leads to less activation of blood cells and coagulation system proteins and thus inhibits production of ROS and proinflammatory cytokines such as IL-6 and MCP-1. Accordingly, the long-term use of an EVOH membrane may reduce oxidative stress and relieve the patients' symptoms of inflammation and help reduce vascular disorders, cardiovascular disease, and death.

References

1 Bonomini M, Pavone B, Sirolli V, et al: Proteomics characterization of protein adsorption onto hemodialysis membranes. J Proteome Res 2006;10:2666–2674.

2 Ishida M: Blood compatibility of Ethylene-vinyl alcohol copolymer dialyzers. Cells 2005;37:30–34 (Japanese).

3 Ito S, Suzuki C, Tsuji T: Platelet activation through interaction with hemodialysis membranes induces neutrophils to produce reactive oxygen species. J Biomed Mater Res 2006;77A:294–303.

4 Sirolli V, Ballone E, Diliberato L, et al: Leukocyte adhesion molecules and leukocyte-platelet interactions during hemodialysis: effect of different synthetic membranes. Int J Artif Organs 1999;22:536–542.

5 Sirolli V, Bonomini M, Di Stante S, et al: Cell activation and cellular-cellular interactions during hemodialysis: effect of dialyzer membrane. Int J Artif Organs 2002;25:529–537.

6 Sato M, Morita H, Ema H, et al: Effect of different dialyzer membranes on cutaneous microcirculation during hemodialysis. Clin Nephrol 2006;66:426–432.

7 Oikawa K, Shimizu M, Mitani S, et al: Influence that EVOH membrane gives to inside and outside of cell transfer of solute and body fluid. The kidneys and dialysis. High Performance Membrane 1997;43(Suppl):83–85 (Japanese).

8 Pertosa G, Simone S, Soccio M, et al: Coagulation cascade activation causes CC chemokine receptor-2 gene expression and mononuclear cell activation in hemodialysis patients. J Am Soc Nephrol 2005;16:2477–2486.

9 Naito H, et al: Effects of various dialysis membranes on the blood clotting system (in Japanese). J Artif Organs 1987;16:763–766.
10 Takemoto Y, et al: Development of techniques to assess the biocompatibility of new synthetic dialysis membranes using intracellular Ca^{2+} dynamics as an index (in Japanese). J Artif Organs 1989;18:1185–1190.
11 Barth RH: Urea modeling and Kt/V: a critical appraisal. Kidney Int 1993;43(suppl 41):S252.
12 Stenvinkel P: Inflammatory and atherosclerotic interactions in the depleted uremic patient. Blood Purif 2001;19:53–61.

Akiyoshi Nakano
EV Plant, Blood Purification Business Unit, Asahi Kasei Kuraray Medical Co. Ltd
4960, Nakagawara-machi, 5-chome, Nobeoka, Miyazaki 882-0031 (Japan)
Tel. +81 982 22 6040 860
E-Mail nakano.ag@om.asahi-kasei.co.jp

Saito A, Kawanishi H, Yamashita AC, Mineshima M (eds): High-Performance Membrane Dialyzers.
Contrib Nephrol. Basel, Karger, 2011, vol 173, pp 172–181

Sustained High-Efficiency Daily Diafiltration Using a Mediator-Adsorbing Membrane (SHEDD-fA) in the Treatment of Patients with Severe Sepsis

Osamu Nishida · Tomoyuki Nakamura · Naohide Kuriyama · Yoshitaka Hara · Miho Yumoto · Yasuyo Shimomura · Kazuhiro Moriyama

Department of Anesthesiology and Critical Care Medicine, Fujita Health University, School of Medicine, Aichi, Japan

Abstract

Sustained high-efficiency daily diafiltration using a mediator-adsorbing membrane (SHEDD-fA) is an effective, intensive modality for sepsis treatment. Here we describe the effectiveness of SHEDD-fA, which makes the best use of three principles: dialysis, filtration and adsorption, for mediator removal in the treatment of severe sepsis. SHEDD-fA was initiated after adequate fluid resuscitation and catecholamine support had been provided. A large ($2.1 m^2$) polymethylmethacrylate membrane dialyzer was placed in the blood circuit. Operation conditions were as follows: blood flow rate 150 ml/min, filtration rate 1,500 ml/h (post-dilution), and dialysate flow rate 300–500 ml/min over 8–12 h daily. 55 consecutive patients with severe sepsis were studied. The following results were obtained: pressure catecholamine index significantly decreased at 3 h after initiation of septic shock, PaO_2/F_{IO2} significantly increased at 1 h after initiation of septic acute respiratory distress syndrome, a significant decrease in interleukin (IL)-6 level for 3 days was observed, and IL-6 was effectively adsorbed in one pass through the filter. The average sequential organ failure assessment score of patients was 10.1 and the mortality at 28 days was 16.4% (46 survived, 9 died). Because SHEDD-fA is an intensive and high-efficiency modality, removal of useful drugs or nutrients may be observed. Despite the fact that removal of useful substances cannot be ignored, we believe that an appropriate stage or timing can be identified so that we can avoid a vicious cycle and use blood purification with effective diffusion, filtration and adsorption. We demonstrate that SHEDD-fA may be an effective, intensive modality for the treatment of patients with severe sepsis and is a possible modality for cytokine modulation therapy.

Despite recent therapeutic improvements, septic shock remains a leading cause of mortality in intensive care patients. Since the early 1990s, experts in the intensive and critical care field have thought that a reduction in cytokines and other mediators including damage-associated molecular patterns (DAMPs) in the blood compartment could reduce mortality; this is because, in these years, these mediators were found to play a pivotal role in severe sepsis and to lead to the development of tissue damage, metabolic acidosis, hypotension and even death [1]. In recent years, some important theories have been put forward as possible explanations for the mediator-targeting blood purification in sepsis. The first one is 'the peak concentration hypothesis', which is the concept of cutting peaks of soluble mediators through blood purification in a non-selective way [2]. The other theories are 'cytokine theory of disease' [3] and 'damage chain reaction' [4]. Harmful stimuli, including pathogens, injury, autoantigens, and necrotic cells, cause tissue damage. Endogenous danger signals are generated and induce a pro-inflammatory cascade by activating Toll-like receptors. In turn, pro-inflammatory mediators are upregulated and trigger further tissue damage leading to increasing DAMP levels. Thus, a vicious cycle is sustained, which warrants the establishment of non-specific elimination of circulating cytokines and other inflammatory mediators by blood purification [5]. The potential value of modifying routine hemofiltration techniques such as high-volume hemofiltration [6] and the use of adsorptive or large-pore-size membranes, such as high cut-off membrane [7], with the aim of removing excess cytokines and treating severe sepsis and septic shock have been discussed [8].

Useful convective removal of mediators from human circulation has not been achieved to date, as many cytokines have a molecular weight of 20–30 kDa, which is below the theoretical cut-off point of the commercial membranes currently used [9]. On the other hand, adsorption has been identified as a major mechanism for cytokine removal both in vitro and in vivo; nevertheless, the membranes used are not specifically designed [10–13].

Sustained high-efficiency daily hemodiafiltration using a mediator-adsorbing membrane (SHEDD-fA) is an effective, intensive modality for sepsis treatment [14]. Here we describe the effectiveness of SHEDD-fA, which makes the best use of three principles: dialysis, filtration and adsorption, for mediator removal, in the treatment of severe sepsis. With regard to the adsorption mechanism, a report from outside Japan has shown that the adsorption reaches saturation in a short time [15]. However, we reconsidered the effective removal of the causative mediators on the basis of the principle of hemofiltration taking an in vitro experiment for the removal of high mobility group box 1 protein (HMGB1) using mediator-adsorbing membrane such as surface-treated polyacrylonitrile (AN69ST) as an example [16].

The aim of the present study was to assess the clinical efficacy of cytokine removal by SHEDD-fA in severe sepsis and septic shock, a typical disease associated with hypercytokinemia in critical care.

Patients and Methods

Patients

All patients with severe sepsis and septic shock who were treated with SHEDD-fA in our intensive care unit during a 1-year period (from July 2005 to June 2006) were investigated retrospectively. Severe sepsis and septic shock were defined according to The American College of Chest Physicians/Society of Critical Care Medicine (ACCP/SCCM) consensus criteria established in 1992.

Measurements

Initial management of circulatory failure began by loading adequate fluid resuscitation. The hemodynamic parameters measured included the systolic blood pressure (SBP), diastolic blood pressure (DBP) and mean arterial pressure (MAP). In cases where MAP was <65 mm Hg, continuous administrations of dopamine (DOA), dobutamine (DOB) and/or norepinephrine (NE) were initiated. Epinephrine (E) was used in septic shock patients who were poorly responsive to DOA or NE. Doses of DOA, DOB, NE and E were recorded (all in μg/kg/min) to compare the total dose of all catecholamines used in different patients by calculating the catecholamine index (CAI) or the pressure catecholamine index (CAIP). CAI and CAIP were calculated with the following formulae [17]:

$$\text{CAI} = \text{DOA dose} + \text{DOB dose} + 100 \times (\text{NE} + \text{E}) \text{ dose } (\mu\text{g/kg/min})$$
$$\text{CAIP} = \text{CAI/MAP}$$

The ratio of the partial pressure of oxygen in arterial blood (PaO_2) to the inspired oxygen fraction (F_{IO2}) was recorded. These parameters were measured before SHEDD-fA treatment and at 1, 3, 6, 24, 48 and 72 h after the start of treatment. Serum interleukin (IL)-6 level was assayed before and three times after SHEDD-fA at 72 h.

IL-6 levels of inlet and outlet of a hemofilter were assayed simultaneously (in order to measure the removal ratio of IL-6 in one pass) in some patients and monocytic human leukocyte antigen (HLA)-DR ratio was assayed in 1 patient. A sequential organ failure assessment (SOFA) score was also assessed for individual patients.

Blood Purification

SHEDD-fA was initiated after adequate fluid resuscitation and catecholamine support had been provided. A polymethylmethacrylate (PMMA) membrane dialyzer (Filtrizer BG-PQ; Toray Medical Co. Ltd, Tokyo, Japan) was placed in the blood circuit. Operation conditions were as follows: blood flow rate (Q_B) 150 ml/min, filtration rate (Q_F) 1,500 ml/h (post-dilution), and dialysate flow rate (Q_D) 300–500 ml/min over 8–12 h daily. The SHEDD-fA system was monitored with a personal bedside console for hemodiafiltration (Nikkiso, Tokyo, Japan). For the purpose of maximizing cytokine adsorption efficiency, we used a large (2.1m^2) PMMA dialyzer. Nafamostat mesilate (Futhan; Torii

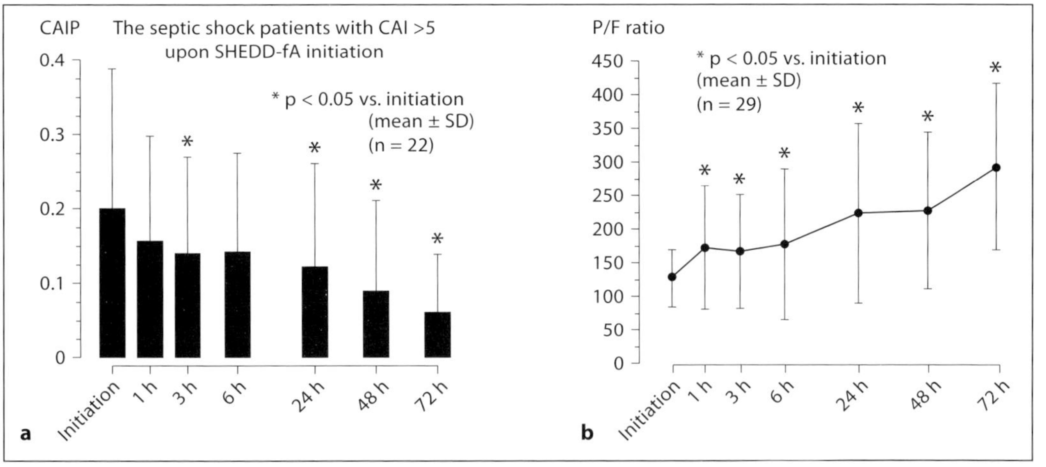

Fig. 1. Effectiveness of SHEDD-fA for septic shock and ARDS. CAI: catecholamine index = DOA dose + DOB dose + 100 × (NE + E) dose (μg/kg/min) (DOA = dopamine, DOB = dobutamine, NE = norepinephrine, E = epinephrine). CAIP: pressure catecholamine index = CAI/mean arterial pressure. P/F ratio = PaO_2/F_{IO2}.

Pharmaceutical Co. Ltd, Tokyo, Japan) was used as anticoagulant, with the dose adjusted to maintain the activated coagulation time of 150 s.

Results

A total of 55 (35 male and 20 female) patients with severe sepsis and septic shock were included in the study. The average age (years) was 66.6 ± 11.2. The SOFA score was 10.11 ± 3.6 (9.8 ± 3.6 survived vs. 11.6 ± 3.3 died, $p = 0.282$, Mann-Whitney U test). The 28-day mortality was 16.4% (46 survived, 9 died).

22 septic shock patients showed CAI >5, despite adequate volume resuscitation. 29 patients were diagnosed with acute respiratory distress syndrome (ARDS) according to the criteria of The American-European Consensus Conference on ARDS in 1994.

Improvement of Hemodynamics

22 septic shock patients showed cardiac index >5, despite adequate volume resuscitation. CAIP significantly increased at 3 h after initiation ($p < 0.05$) and decreased day by day for 3 days ($p < 0.05$) (fig. 1a).

Improvement of PaO_2/F_{IO2}

29 septic ARDS patients showed PaO_2/F_{IO2} <200. The average PaO_2/F_{IO2} ratio increased at 1 h ($p < 0.05$) after the start of treatment, and improved continuously for 3 days ($p < 0.05$) (fig. 1b).

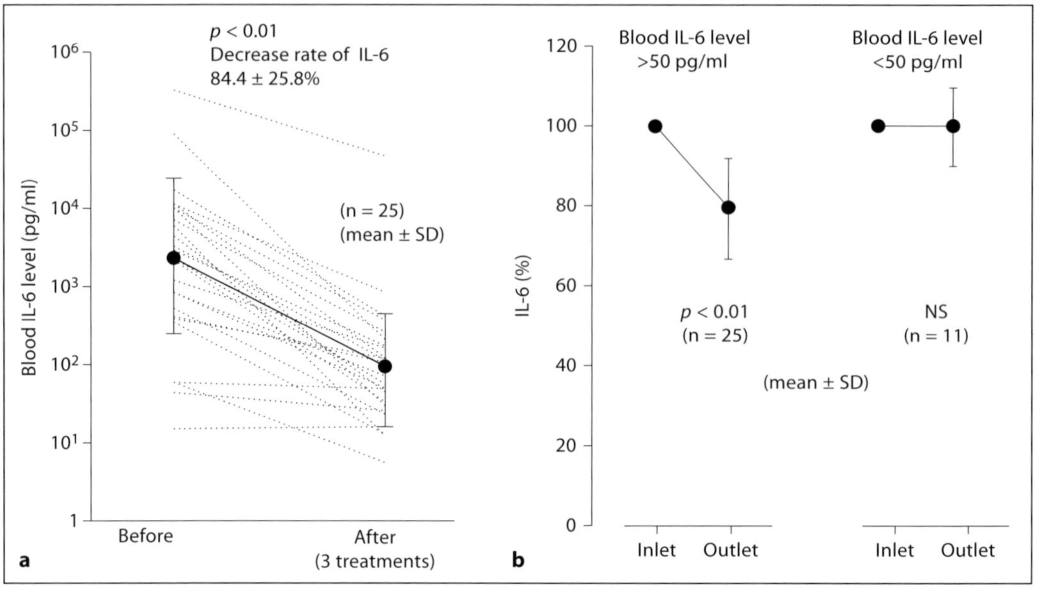

Fig. 2. Decreased IL-6 in blood and removal ratio in one pass through hemofilter.

IL-6 Blood Level

In 25 patients out of 55, IL-6 blood levels before initiation were analyzed. A significant decrease in blood IL-6 level after three SHEDD-fA treatments during 3 days was observed. The average IL-6 level decreased for 3 days ($p < 0.01$) and the decreasing rate was 84.4 ± 25.8% (fig. 2a). Furthermore, we showed a change in blood IL-6 concentration from the pre- to the post-hemofilter point (fig. 2b). The concentration of IL-6 decreased at the exit of the column by 21.0 ± 13.4% in the patients who showed initial IL-6 levels >50 pg/ml, showing that IL-6 was effectively removed in one pass through the hemofilter. On the other hand, the patients who showed initial IL-6 levels <50 pg/ml did not show a decrease (fig. 2b). The results were that 13 of 16 patients who showed IL-6 levels >10,000 pg/ml before treatment survived. Moreover, the depressed monocytic HLA-DR ratio was improved from 40.6 to 51.9% in 1 typical immunoparalytic case (fig. 3).

Discussion

We demonstrated the CAIP decrease for septic shock, PaO_2/F_{IO2} increase for septic ARDS, IL-6 decrease, and one pass IL-6 removal through the filter. The average SOFA score of patients was 10.1 and the mortality at 28 days was 16.4%. In 1 case, there was a possibility to improve immunoparalysis from the increase of monocytic HLA-DR ratio. These findings may be rational from the

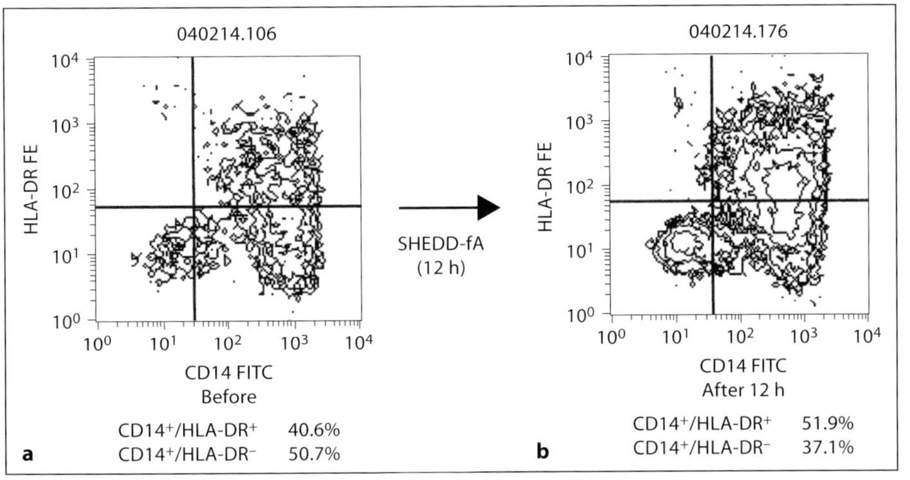

Fig. 3. Change of HLA-DR antigen before (**a**) and after (**b**) SHEDD-fA.

viewpoints of the peak concentration hypothesis [2], cytokine theory of disease [3] and damage chain reaction [4].

Many water-soluble mediators with pro- and anti-inflammatory action play a strategic role in sepsis. In intensive care medicine, however, blocking of single mediator has not led to a measurable improvement in patients with sepsis. This outcome has provided the rationale for non-specific elimination of circulating cytokines, not only pro-inflammatory mediators but anti-inflammatory mediators, and other inflammatory mediators to the level which is dealt with the self-defenses induced by a nearly normal immunohomeostasis treated by our high efficient blood purification. SHEDD-fA also showed the possibility to improve immunoparalysis from the depressed monocytic HLA-DR ratio by reducing anti-inflammatory mediators.

SHEDD-fA, which resembles sustained low-efficiency daily dialysis (SLEDD) to some extent, is not merely a hybrid therapy but a high-efficiency, intensive and intermittent modality with effective setting (diffusion, filtration and adsorption) for 10 h/day to break a vicious cycle by removing cytokines efficiently from the blood. SLEDD is defined as the hybrid modality between CRRT and IRRT; Q_B, Q_D is the range within 100–300 ml/min for 8–12 h/day, with an advantage of simple method, cost effectiveness, low incidence of complication and giving the time for inspection outside the intensive care unit [18]. On the other hand, SHEDD-fA is not a mere hybrid therapy but a high-efficiency, intensive, intermittent modality: blood flow rate (Q_B) 150 ml/min, filtration rate (Q_F) 1,500 ml/h (post-dilution) and dialysate flow rate (Q_D) 300–500 ml/min with large-size mediator-adsorbing membrane over 8–12 h daily or prolonged according to the patient's severity. As high-efficiency blood purification

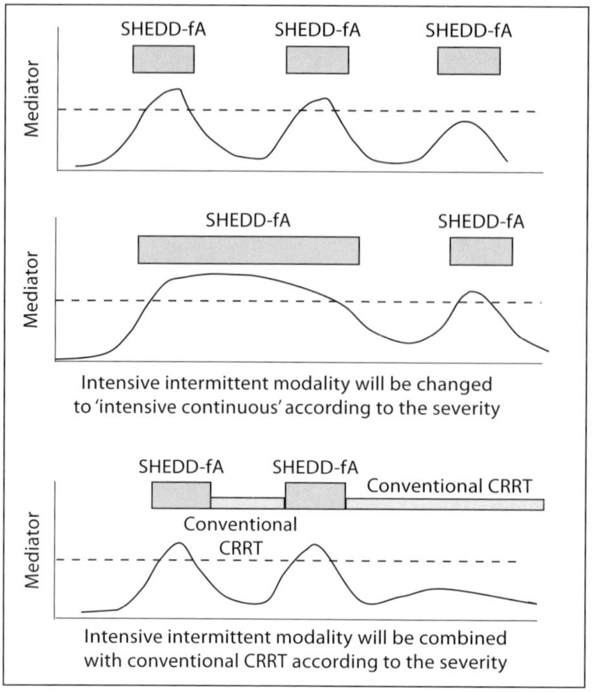

Fig. 4. Concept of SHEDD-fA. Dashed line shows the limit of mediators level which is dealt with the self-defenses induced by a nearly normal immunohomeostasis.

techniques, high-volume hemofiltration and high-flow-volume hemodiafiltration, such as short-term high-volume hemofiltration, are available. Taking into account excess removal of useful substances due to the high efficiency, use of an intermittent modality may have advantages of restoration considering the patient's circadian rhythm and allowing the time needed for useful substances to act, besides its advantage of simplicity.

This modality is thought to be changed to, for example, continuous modality or combination modality with conventional CRRT according the patient condition, because SHEDD-fA is designed to break the vicious cycle by reducing cytokines efficiently from the blood (fig. 4). Continuous modality has been the initiative in acute blood purification in critical care. Now is the time to reconsider the modality of blood purification in critical care according to the severity of disease such as a ventilator setting.

With regard to the adsorption mechanism, a report from outside Japan has shown that the adsorption reaches saturation in a short time [15]. However, we showed the effectiveness of adsorption by in vitro experiment for the removal of HMGB1 [16, 19], which is a novel therapeutic target for sepsis [20]. Among the hemofilters, AN69ST showed the highest capacity to adsorb HMGB1; it adsorbed nearly 100 μg of HMGB1 in the initial 60 min and showed a markedly high clearance rate of 60.8 ± 5.0 ml/min at 15 min for the solution flow of 100 ml/min. PMMA membrane showed rates of 25.8 ± 4.8, polysulfone membrane and high cut-off filter showed rates of 7.0 ± 9.1 and 18.7 ± 4.4 ml/min, respectively. Furthermore, HMGB1 of 100 μg was adsorbed by AN69ST in the initial 60 min and then added six times by 100 μg for every hour, and 700 μg of HMGB1 in total were adsorbed by the same filter (published in Japanese). No saturation phenomenon was observed. Therefore, we concluded that continuous hemofiltration using the AN69ST membrane is a promising approach for HMGB1-related sepsis.

However, we should discuss the questions that inevitably arise concerning this approach. SHEDD-fA may induce underdosing of antibiotics [21]. Sufficient doses of antibiotics should be administered if possible using the therapeutic drag monitoring. Nutrition status such as that of amino acids may be compromised [22]. We clinically start early enteral nutrition inserting a feeding tube over Treitz ligament into intestinal jejunum. Enteral nutrition would be better tolerated than parenteral nutrition in terms of removal by blood purification.

In some cases, a drop of systolic blood pressure within 30 min from initiation was observed. Fluid supplementation or transit increase of catecholamine improves hemodynamics gradually in many cases. We call this phenomenon 'initial drop', which is thought to be initial removal of catecholamine from blood.

Patients who showed elevated BUN may develop dialysis disequilibrium syndrome when first receiving intensive blood purification. Decreasing the removal efficiency for first-time solute should be considered according to the data of blood osmolarity in such cases.

Finally, we concluded that the careful use of SHEDD-fA may be an effective, intensive modality for the treatment of patients with severe sepsis and is a possible modality for cytokine modulation therapy.

Closing Remarks

A simple comparison of dose for blood purification seems to be inadequate. Moreover, note that there has been no actual discussion or consideration as to the hemofilter characteristics. Furthermore, at present, even the target mediators have not been clarified sufficiently, in terms of which substances and how much we should remove according to the severity or type of critical illness. We hypothesized that it may be possible to contribute to the recovery from illness by breaking the vicious cycle of pathogens or mediators. Despite the fact that the removal of useful substances cannot be ignored, we believe that an appropriate stage or timing can be identified so that we can break the vicious cycle using blood purification with effective diffusion, filtration and adsorption [23].

However, when should we start, when should we stop and how much should the dose be? The time may come soon when the dose and modality can be changed according to the patient condition, like the changes of ventilator settings that are adapted to the patient condition.

References

1 Rittirsch D, Flierl MA, Ward PA: Harmful molecular mechanisms in sepsis. Nat Rev Immunol 2008;8:776–787.

2 Ronco C, Tetta C, Mariano F, et al: Interpreting the mechanisms of continuous renal replacement therapy in sepsis: the peak concentration hypothesis. Artif Organs 2003;27:792–801.

3 Tracey KJ: Physiology and immunology of the cholingergic anti-inflammatory pathway. J Clin Invest 2007;117:289–296.

4 Piccinini AM, Midwood KS: DAMPening inflammation by modulating TLR signalling. Mediators Inflamm 2010;pii:672395.

5 Hirasawa H: Indications for blood purification in critical care. Contrib Nephrol. Basel, Karger, 2010, vol 166, pp 21–30.

6 Honoré PM, Jamez J, Wauthier M, et al: Prospective evaluation of short-term high-volume isovolemic hemofiltration on the hemodynamic course and outcome in patients with intractable circulatory failure resulting from septic shock. Crit Care Med 2000;28:3581–3587.

7 Morgera S, Haase M, Kuss T, et al: Pilot study on the effects of high cut-off hemofiltration on the need for norepinephrine in septic patients with acute renal failure. Crit Care Med 2006;34:2099–2104.

8 Ronco C, Kellum JA, Bellomo R, et al: Potential interventions in sepsis-related acute kidney injury. Clin J Am Soc Nephrol 2008;3:531–544.

9 Moriyama K, Soejima Y: Continuous hemodiafiltration using PMMA membrane: clinical efficacy and its mechanisms. Contrib Nephrol. Basel, Karger, 1999, vol 125, pp 222–232.

10 Nakada TA, Oda S, Matsuda K, et al: Continuous hemodiafiltration with PMMA hemofilter in the treatment of patients with septic shock. Mol Med 2008;14:257–263.

11 Chanard J, Lavaud S, Paris B, et al: Assessment of heparin binding to the AN69ST hemodialysis membrane. I. Preclinical studies. ASAIO J 2005;51:342–347.

12 Gong D, Zhang P, Ji D, et al: Improvement of immune dysfunction in patients with severe acute pancreatitis by high-volume hemofiltration: a preliminary report. Int J Artif Organs 2010;33:22–29.

13 Rimmele T, Assadi A, Cattenoz M, et al: High-volume haemofiltration with a new haemofiltration membrane having enhanced adsorption properties in septic pigs. Nephrol Dial Transplant 2009;24:421–427.

14 Nishida O, Nakamura T, Kuriyama N, et al: Sustained high-efficiency daily diafiltration using a cytokine-adsorbing membrane in the treatment of patients with severe sepsis. Crit Care 2011;15(suppl 1):115.

15 De Vriese AS, Colardyn FA, Philippé JJ, et al : Cytokine removal during continuous hemofiltration in septic patients. J Am Soc Nephrol 1999;10:846–853.

16 Yumoto M, Nishida O, Moriyama K, et al: In vitro evaluation of HMGB1 removal with various membranes for continuous hemofiltration. Crit Care 2011;5(suppl 1):114.

17 Cruz DN, Antonelli M, Fumagalli R et al : Early use of polymyxin B hemoperfusion in abdominal septic shock. JAMA 2009;301:2445–2452.

18 Fliser D, Kielstein JT: Technology Insight: treatment of renal failure in the intensive care unit with extended dialysis. Nat Clin Pract Nephrol 2006;2:32–39.

19 Yumoto M, Nishida O, Moriyama K, et al: In vitro evaluation of high mobility group box 1 protein removal with various membranes for continuous hemofiltration. Ther Apher Dial 2011 (in press).

20 Wang H, Ward MF, Sama AE: Novel HMGB1-inhibiting therapeutic agents for experimental sepsis. Shock 2009;32:348–357.
21 Bouman CSC: Antimicrobial dosing strategies in critically ill patients with acute kidney injury and high-dose continuous veno-venous hemofiltration. Curr Opin Crit Care 2008;14:654–659.
22 Schiffl H: The dark side of high-intensity renal replacement therapy of acute kidney injury in critically ill patients. Int Urol Nephrol 2010;42:435–440.
23 Joannes-Boyau O, Honoré PM, Boer W, et al: Are the synergistic effects of high-volume haemofiltration and enhanced adsorption the missing key in sepsis modulation? Nephrol Dial Transplant 2009;24:354–357.

Osamu Nishida, MD, PhD
Department of Anesthesiology and Critical Care Medicine
Fujita Health University School of Medicine
1-98 Dengakugakubo, Kutsukake-cho, Toyoake, Aichi 470-1192 (Japan)
E-Mail nishida@fujita-hu.ac.jp

Saito A, Kawanishi H, Yamashita AC, Mineshima M (eds): High-Performance Membrane Dialyzers.
Contrib Nephrol. Basel, Karger, 2011, vol 173, pp 182–190

Comparison of Efficacy between Continuous Hemodiafiltration with a PMMA High-Performance Membrane Dialyzer and a PAN Membrane Hemofilter in the Treatment of Septic Shock Patients with Acute Renal Failure

Kenichi Matsuda · Takeshi Moriguchi · Norikazu Harii · Masahiko Yanagisawa · Daiki Harada · Hisanori Sugawara

Department of Emergency and Critical Care Medicine, University of Yamanashi School of Medicine, Yamanashi, Japan

Abstract

The aim of this study was to investigate whether continuous hemodiafiltration (CHDF) with a high-performance membrane dialyzer made of polymethylmethacrylate (PMMA-CHDF) in the treatment of septic shock patients with acute renal failure (ARF) is clinically relevant. 30 patients were treated with PMMA-CHDF. 13 patients treated with CHDF used a hemofilter made of polyacrylonitrile membrane (PAN-CHDF). Systolic blood pressure significantly increased in the PMMA-CHDF group following 24 h of treatment ($p < 0.01$), whereas it did not improve in the PAN-CHDF group. Urine volume significantly increased in the PMMA-CHDF group following 24 h of treatment which was more than in the PAN-CHDF group ($p < 0.05$). 28-day survival was 83.3% in the PMMA-CHDF group and 30.8% in the PAN-CHDF group, respectively ($p < 0.01$). We can assume that PMMA-CHDF in the treatment of septic shock patients with ARF is clinically relevant.

In 2000, a study by Ronco et al. [1] published in *The Lancet* was the first large prospective randomized controlled study of blood purification for critically ill patients. In the study, high-volume continuous hemofiltration (CHF) could change survival of critically ill patients. Honore et al. [2] insisted that a 'big bang' of clinical blood purification would take place when the study was published and that it was believed by many that the use of hemofiltration at a certain dose would change the survival rate in intensive care since that big bang. However, high-volume CHF has not been widely adopted in the world. Bellomo [3], one of the study's authors, assumed some reasons in a commentary such as the necessity of high blood flow for getting a high filtrate and high cost for the high volume of substitute fluid. On the other hand, continuous hemodiafiltration with a high-performance membrane dialyzer made of polymethylmethacrylate membrane-continuous hemodiafiltration (PMMA-CHDF) removes cytokines from the bloodstream mainly by adsorption, rather than convection and diffusion [4–8]. Therefore, PMMA-CHDF does not require a high blood flow and a large volume of sterile fluid. From the viewpoint of safety and cost, it becomes clear that PMMA-CHDF is superior to high-volume CHF in the treatment of critically ill patients with hypercytokinemia.

The aim of the present study was to investigate whether PMMA-CHDF in the treatment of septic shock patients with acute renal failure (ARF) is clinically relevant compared with CHDF with a hemofilter made of polyacrylonitrile membrane (PAN-CHDF), which is not able to remove enough humoral mediators from the bloodstream under conventional operational conditions [1–3, 9].

Materials and Methods

Patients

Forty-three consecutive septic shock patients with ARF admitted to the intensive care unit (ICU) at the University of Yamanashi Hospital and who received critical care including CHDF in the period from January 2000 to September 2010 were entered in this study. 13 consecutive patients were treated with PAN-CHDF between January 2000 and September 2005 (PAN-CHDF group). 30 consecutive patients were treated with PMMA-CHDF between October 2005 and September 2010 (PMMA-CHDF group).

These patients fulfilled the following criteria: (a) Patients exhibited septic shock with ARF at ICU admission or developed it within 24 h after ICU admission. Septic shock was defined according to the American College of Chest Physicians/Society of Critical Care Medicine (ACCP/SCCM) consensus criteria established in 1992 [10]. ARF was defined by a serum creatinine level >3.5 mg/dl or a urine output <500 ml/day despite fluid resuscitation and furosemide administration [11]. (b) PMMA-CHDF or PAN-CHDF was initiated within 24 h after development of ARF.

The exclusion criteria for the present study were: (a) septic shock with ARF developing 24 h after ICU admission; (b) an age of 18 years or younger; (c) severe heart failure (New York Heart Association: NYHA class IV), and (d) patients died within 24 h after ICU admission.

Operational Conditions of CHDF

Vascular access was provided by placing a 12-Fr flexible triple-lumen catheter (Blood Access Triple-Lumen Catheter; Arrow International Inc., Reading, Pa., USA) in the internal jugular vein or the femoral vein.

Operation of the hemodiafiltration system was monitored with a personal bedside console (JUN-500; Ube Medical Co. Ltd, Tokyo, Japan). Nafamostat mesilate (Futhan; Torii Pharmaceutical Co. Ltd, Tokyo, Japan) was used as anticoagulant, with the dose adjusted to maintain an activated coagulation time of 150–170 s.

In the PAN-CHDF group the material of the hemofilter was polyacrylonitrile. The membrane area of the hemofilter was 1.0 m^2 (Panflo APF-10S; Asahi Kasei Kuraray Medical Co. Ltd, Tokyo, Japan). Blood flow rate was 80–100 ml/min. Dialyzate flow rate and filtrate flow rate were 500 and 300 ml/h, respectively.

On the other hand, in the PMMA-CHDF group, material of the high-performance membrane dialyzer was polymethylmethacrylate. The membrane area of the dialyzer was 2.1 m^2 (Filtryzer BK-2.1P; Toray Medical Co. Ltd, Tokyo, Japan). Blood flow rate was 100–120 ml/min and dialyzate flow rate and filtrate flow rate were 1,000 and 300–600 ml/h, respectively.

Measurements

On admission to the ICU, the severity of septic shock patients with ARF was evaluated according to the acute physiology and chronic health evaluation (APACHE) II score [12] and sequential organ failure assessment (SOFA) score [11] before treatment. Changes in systolic blood pressure (SBP) and dose of catecholamine following 24 h of treatment were compared between the PAN-CHDF group and PMMA-CHDF group. The dose of catecholamine was calculated with the following equation as catecholamine index (CAI):

$$\text{CAI} = \text{dopamine} + \text{dobutamine} + \text{norepinephrine} \times 100\ (\mu\text{g/kg/min})$$

Changes in water balances per 8 h from 8 h before initiation of CHDF to the following 24 h of treatment with CHDF were compared between the two groups. Urine volumes following 24 h of treatment were compared between the two groups. 28-day survivals were also compared between the groups.

Statistical Analysis

Values are the mean ± SD. The demographic and physiologic variables of septic shock patients with ARF before CHDF treatment were compared statistically between the groups by χ^2 test and two-tailed paired t test. Changes in SBP, CAI and water balances were compared statistically between the groups by repeated measure ANOVA and each value was compared statistically by two-tailed paired t test. Urine volumes were compared statistically by two-tailed paired t test. p values <0.05 were considered statistically significant. A computer software package (GraphPad Prism 4; GraphPad Software Inc., San Diego, Calif., USA) was used for all statistical analyses.

Results

The demographic and physiologic variables of septic shock patients with ARF before treatment are shown in table 1. The average ages in the PAN-CHDF and PMMA-CHDF group were 61.4 ± 12.1 and 63.9 ± 12.3, respectively. APACHE II scores were 26.8 ± 8.3 and 29.0 ± 6.7, respectively. Predicted death rates calculated from the APACHE II score were 58.1 ± 24.5 and 64.4 ± 19.6%, respectively.

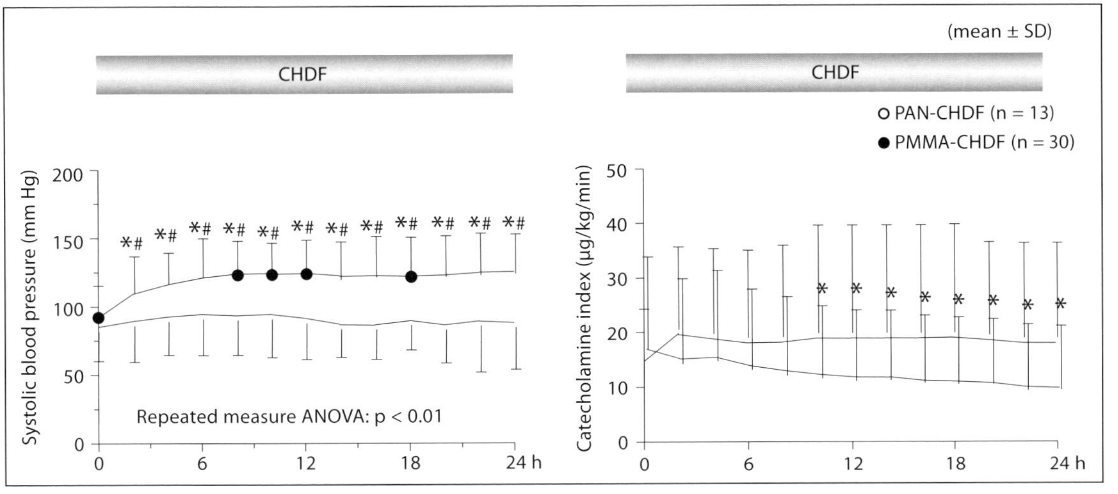

Fig. 1. Changes in SBP and CAI in the treatment with CHDF between the PAN-CHDF group and PMMA-CHDF group (CAI: dopamine + dobutamine + norepinephrine × 100 (µg/kg/min). * $p < 0.05$ compared to the value before CHDF; # $p < 0.05$ compared between the groups.

Table 1. Demographic and physiologic variables of septic shock patients with ARF before treatment (mean ± SD)

	PAN-CHDF group (n = 13)	PMMA-CHDF group (n = 30)	p value
Age, years	61.4 ± 12.1	63.9 ± 12.3	ns
Male/female	11/2	19/11	ns
Background of sepsis			
Peritonitis	9	17	
Pneumonia	2	8	
Others	2	5	
APACHE II score	26.8 ± 8.3	29.0 ± 6.7	ns
Predicted death rate, %	58.1 ± 24.5	64.4 ± 19.6	ns
SOFA score	11.8 ± 3.9	13.0 ± 3.7	ns

SOFA scores were 11.8 ± 3.9 and 13.0 ± 3.7, respectively. There were no significant differences in the pretreatment clinical profiles between the two groups.

Comparison of changes in SBP and CAI in the treatment with CHDF between the PAN-CHDF group and PMMA-CHDF group is shown in figure 1. There was a significant difference of the changes in SBP per 2 h following 24 h of treatment in the septic shock patients with ARF between the two groups ($p < 0.01$). In the

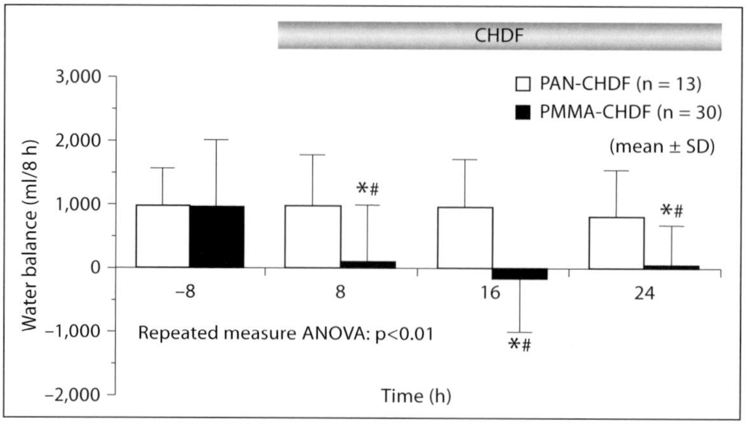

Fig. 2. Changes in water balances per 8 h from 8 h before initiation of CHDF in the following 24 h of treatment with CHDF were compared between the PAN-CHDF group and PMMA-CHDF group. * $p < 0.05$ compared to the value before CHDF; # $p < 0.05$ compared between the groups.

PAN-CHDF group, SBP did not increase after the initiation of PAN-CHDF even if CAI increased. On the other hand, in the PMMA-CHDF group, SBP significantly increased after the initiation of PMMA-CHDF even if CAI decreased.

Comparison of changes in water balance of each 8 h from 8 h before initiation of CHDF to 24 h after treatment of CHDF between the PAN-CHDF group and PMMA-CHDF group is shown in figure 2. There was a significant difference of the changes in water balances per 8 h from 8 h before initiation of CHDF to the following 24 h of treatment with CHDF compared between the two groups ($p < 0.01$). In the PAN-CHDF group, fluid administration should be continued after the initiation of PAN-CHDF in contrast to the PMMA-CHDF group.

Urine volumes following 24 h of treatment in the PAN-CHDF and PMMA-CHDF group were 610 ± 710 and 1,490 ± 1,420 ml/day, respectively. There was a significant difference of urine volume between the two groups ($p < 0.05$).

Comparison of cumulative survival of the septic shock patients with ARF between the PAN-CHDF group and PMMA-CHDF group is shown in figure 3. The cumulative survival in the PMMA-CHDF group was significantly higher than that in the PAN-CHDF group ($p < 0.01$). The 28-day survival rate of septic shock patients with ARF in the PMMA-CHDF group and PAN-CHDF group were 83.3 and 30.8%, respectively.

Discussion

In this study it was revealed that PMMA-CHDF can increase SBP in septic shock patients with ARF for 24 h (fig. 1) and that the efficacy of PMMA-CHDF for SBP

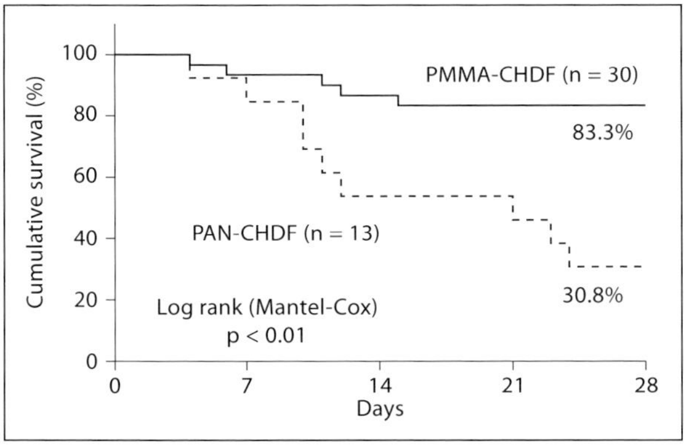

Fig. 3. Comparison of cumulative survival of septic shock patients with ARF between the PAN-CHDF group and PMMA-CHDF group.

is not due to fluid loading (fig. 2). We have reported previously that PMMA-CHDF exhibited a higher capacity to remove cytokines than PAN-CHDF and that blood cytokine levels in critically ill patients with hypercytokinemia were significantly decreased after PMMA-CHDF treatment [4, 5, 13]. Based on these findings it is possible to consider that the efficacy of PMMA-CHDF for SBP is due to not fluid loading but cytokine modulation with PMMA-CHDF; even the blood level of cytokines was not measured in this study.

We have also reported previously that the high capacity for cytokine removal of PMMA-CHDF was principally ascribable to adsorption of cytokines to the hemofilter membrane rather than convection and diffusion, and that the capacity of cytokine adsorption of PMMA-CHDF had been kept for more than 24 h [4, 13]. It was reported that PAN membrane also has the capacity of cytokine adsorption but that the capacity was not enough [14]. This led to a necessary change of the PAN hemofilter every 3 h if the capacity of cytokine adsorption of PAN membrane applied to the removal of cytokine [14]. Based on the findings that the PMMA membrane has a capacity of cytokine adsorption superior to that of PAN membrane, it is possible to be elucidated that SBP had increased for 24 h after the initiation of PMMA-CHDF (fig. 1).

Since the 1980s, it has been advocated [15–17] that removal of the humoral mediators with blood purifications was useful in the treatment of sepsis and septic multiple organ failure. Although the removal of several causative mediators with blood purifications had been demonstrated in animal and human studies, the lack of the standardization and large randomized clinical trials in this area had made the role of blood purification as a mediator remover in sepsis and other critical conditions controversial [18–20].

Recently, the efficacy of cytokine modulation with blood purification in the treatment of critically ill patients has been widely accepted [2, 9, 21–24].

Simultaneously, various cytokine removal technologies have been applied to the treatment of critically ill patients with hypercytokinemia, such as severe sepsis and septic shock [14, 25–30]. In these studies, many investigations reported that the various types of blood purification therapy could improve the survival of critically ill patients with hypercytokinemia from about 30% to about 60%. However, PMMA-CHDF could improve the survival from 30% to about 80%, and even the APACHE II and SOFA scores of the patients were extremely high (fig. 3) [5, 8]. From the viewpoint of survival, it is possible to conclude that PMMA-CHDF is superior to other blood purifications in the treatment of critically ill patients with hypercytokinemia.

The present study had some limitations: (1) it was not designed as a prospective randomized study; (2) the sample size was small; (3) it was performed over a long period of time, and (4) it was performed in a single center. A randomized, controlled trial with a larger sample size is needed to confirm the clinical efficacy of PMMA-CHDF in treating septic shock patients with ARF; it even became difficult to perform PAN-CHDF in critically ill patients in our institution for ethical reasons after this study.

In conclusion, PMMA-CHDF could significantly increase SBP and urine volume in septic shock patients with ARF. In addition, PMMA-CHDF could dramatically improve the survival rate in septic shock patients with ARF. Therefore, it can be assumed that PMMA-CHDF in the treatment of septic shock patients with ARF is clinically relevant.

References

1 Ronco C, Bellomo R, Homel P, Brendolan A, Dan M, Piccinni P, La Greca G: Effects of different doses in continuous veno-venous haemofiltration on outcomes of acute renal failure: a prospective randomized trial. Lancet 2000;355:26–30.

2 Honore PM, Joannes-Boyau O, Merson L, Boer W, Piette V, Galloy AC, Janvier G: The big bang of hemofiltration: the beginning of a new era in the third millennium for extracorporeal blood purification! Int J Artif Organs 2006;29:649–659.

3 Bellomo R: Do we know the optimal dose for renal replacement therapy in the intensive care unit? Kidney Int 2006;70:1202–1204.

4 Hirasawa H, Oda S, Matsuda K: Continuous hemodiafiltration with cytokine-adsorbing hemofilter in the treatment of severe sepsis and septic shock. Contrib Nephrol. Basel, Karger, 2007, vol 156, pp 365–370.

5 Nakada T, Oda S, Matsuda K, Sadahiro T, Nakamura M, Abe R, Hirasawa H: Continuous hemodiafiltration with PMMA hemofilter in the treatment of patients with septic shock. Mol Med 2008;14:257–263.

6 Matsuda K, Moriguchi T, Harii N, Goto J: Comparison of efficacy between continuous hemodiafiltration with a PMMA membrane hemofilter and a PAN membrane hemofilter in the treatment of a patient with septic acute renal failure. Transfus Apher Sci 2009;40:49–53.

7 Matsuda K, Moriguchi T, Oda S, Hirasawa H: Efficacy of continuous hemodiafiltration with a cytokine-adsorbing hemofilter in the treatment of acute respiratory distress syndrome. Contrib Nephrol. Basel, Karger, 2010, vol 166, pp 83–92.

8 Nakamura M, Oda S, Sadahiro T, Hirayama Y, Watanabe E, Tateishi Y, Nakada TA, Hirasawa H: Treatment of severe sepsis and septic shock by CHDF using a PMMA membrane hemofilter as a cytokine modulator. Contrib Nephrol. Basel, Karger, 2010, vol 166, pp 73–82.
9 Honore PM, Joannes-Boyaub O, Gressensa B: Blood and plasma treatments: the rationale of high-volume hemofiltration. Contrib Nephrol. Basel, Karger, 2007, vol 156, pp 387–395.
10 Members of the American College of Chest Physicians/Society of Critical Care Medicine Consensus Conference Committee: American College of Chest Physicians/Society of Critical Care Medicine Consensus Conference: Definitions for sepsis and organ failure and guidelines for the use of innovative therapies in sepsis. Crit Care Med 1992;20:864–874.
11 Vincent JL, de Mendonca A, Cantraine F, Moreno R, Takala J, Suter P, Sprung CL, Colardyn F, Blecher S: Use of the SOFA score to assess the incidence of organ dysfunction/failure in intensive care units: results of a multicenter, prospective study. Crit Care Med 1998;26:1793–1800.
12 Knaus WA, Draper EA, Wagner DP, Zimmerman JE: APACHE II: a severity of disease classification system. Crit Care Med 1985;13:818–829.
13 Matsuda K, Hirasawa H, Oda S, Shiga H, Nakanishi K: Current topics on cytokine removal technologies. Ther Apher 2001;5:306–314.
14 Haase M, Silvester W, Uchino S, Goldsmith D, Davenport P, Tipping P, Boyce N, Bellomo R: A pilot study of high-adsorption hemofiltration in human septic shock. Int J Artif Organs 2007;30:108–117.
15 Hirasawa H, Odaka M, Kobayashi H, Soeda K, Kobayashi S, Murotani N, Ito Y, Isono K: Hemopurification in the treatment of patients with multiple organ failure; in Nose Y, Kjellstrand C, Ivanovich P (eds): Progress in Artificial Organs, 1985. Cleveland, ISAO Press, 1986, pp 730–734.
16 Stein B, Pfenninger E, Gruenert A, Schmitz JE, Hudde M: Influence of continuous haemofiltration on haemodynamics and central blood volume in experimental endotoxic shock. Intensive Care Med 1990;16:494–499.
17 Hirasawa H, Sugai T, Ohtake Y, Oda S, Matsuda K, Kitamura N: Blood purification for prevention and treatment of multiple organ failure. World J Surg 1996;20:482–486.
18 Kellum JA: Immunomodulation in sepsis: the role of hemofiltration. Minerva Anestesiol 1999;65:410–418.
19 De Vriese AS, Vanholder RC, Pascual M, Lameire NH, Colardyn FA: Can inflammatory cytokines be removed efficiency by continuous renal replacement therapies? Intensive Care Med 1999;25:903–910.
20 Rogiers P: Hemofiltration treatment for sepsis: is it time for controlled trials? Kidney Int 1999;72(suppl):S99–S103.
21 Ronco C, Bonello M, Bordonia V, Ricci Z, D'Intini V, Bellomo R, Levin NW: Extracorporeal therapies in non-renal disease: treatment of sepsis and the peak concentration hypothesis. Blood Purif 2004;22:164–174.
22 Honore PM, Joannes-Boyau O: High-volume hemofiltration in sepsis: a comprehensive review of rationale, clinical applicability, potential indications and recommendations for future research. Int J Artif Organs 2004;27:1077–1082.
23 Di Carlo JV, Alexander SR: Hemofiltration for cytokine-driven illnesses: the mediator delivery hypothesis. Int J Artif Organs 2005;28:777–786.
24 Hirasawa H: Indications for blood purification in critical care. Contrib Nephrol. Basel, Karger, 2010, vol 166, pp 21–30.
25 Busund R, Koukline V, Utrobin U, Nedashkovsky E: Plasmapheresis in severe sepsis and septic shock: a prospective, randomised, controlled trial. Intensive Care Med 2002;28:1434–1439.
26 Piccinni P, Dan M, Barbacini S, Carraro R, Lieta E, Marafon S, Zamperetti N, Brendolan A, D'Intini V, Tetta C, Bellomo R, Ronco C: Early isovolaemic haemofiltration in oliguric patients with septic shock. Intensive Care Med 2006;32:80–86.

27 Saudan P, Niederberger M, Seigneux SD, Romand J, Pugin J, Perneger T, Martin PY: Adding a dialysis dose to continuous hemofiltration increases survival in patients with acute renal failure. Kidney Int 2006;70:1312–1317.
28 House AA, Ronco C: Extracorporeal blood purification in sepsis and sepsis-related acute kidney injury. Blood Purif 2008;26:30–35.
29 Joannidis M: Continuous renal replacement therapy in sepsis and multisystem organ failure. Semin Dial 2009;22:160–64.
30 Schefold JC, Hasper D, Jörres A: Organ crosstalk in critically ill patients: hemofiltration and immunomodulation in sepsis. Blood Purif 2009;28:116–123.

Kenichi Matsuda
Department of Emergency and Critical Care Medicine
University of Yamanashi School of Medicine
1110 Shimokato Chuo, Yamanashi 409-3898 (Japan)
Tel. +81 55 273 9812, E-Mail matsudak@yamanashi.ac.jp

Saito A, Kawanishi H, Yamashita AC, Mineshima M (eds): High-Performance Membrane Dialyzers.
Contrib Nephrol. Basel, Karger, 2011, vol 173, pp 191–195

Commercially Available High-Performance Membrane Dialyzers and Several Special Kinds on the Japanese Market (as of April 30, 2011)

A.C. Yamashita

Department of Human and Environmental Science, School of Engineering, Shonan Institute of Technology, Tsujido-Nishikaigan, Fujisawa, Kanagawa, Japan

A.C. Yamashita
Department of Human and Environmental Science
School of Engineering, Shonan Institute of Technology
1-1-25 Tsujido-Nishikaigan, Fujisawa, Kanagawa 251-8511 (Japan)
Tel./Fax +81 466 300234, E-Mail yama@la.shonan-it.ac.jp

No.	Maker	Japanese brand name	Main material of the membrane	Surface area A_o, m^2	Clearance, ml/min^{B,C}			Class according to the Japanese reimburse-ment system	Ultrafiltration coefficient $k_{UF}^{B,D}$ ml/h/mm Hg	Albumin loss		
					urea nitro-gen	creati-nine	β_2-MG			targeted value per 4-hour clinical treatment, g	in vitro 4-hour dialysis experiment, g	*s.c.* @ XXX min (Q_B = XXX, Q_F = YY, ml/min) [–]
1	Fresenius Medical Care Japan KK	FX 140	PS	1.4	198	182	49	IV	49	0.1–0.3	NA	NA
		Notes: Aqueous solution was used for measuring clearances of urea nitrogen and creatinine at Q_F = 0 ml/min/m^2 and bovine plasma was used for β_2-microgloulin clearance at Q_F = 10 ml/min/m^2, and bovine blood was used for UFR (Ht 32 ± 2%, TP 6.0 ± 0.5 g/dl)										
2		FX-S 140	PS	1.4	196	182	68	V	50	2.0–3.0	NA	NA
3	Asahi Kasei-Kuraray Medical Co. Ltd	APS-15EA	PS	1.5	197	197	73	V	56	1.5	NA	0.01 @ 60 min (Q_B = 200, Q_F = 15 ml/min)
		Notes: Clearance (urea nitrogen, creatinine) in aqueous solution, TMP = 0 kPa (0 mm Hg)Ultrafiltration coefficient with bovine blood s.c. (albumin) with bovine plasma										
4		APS-15SA	PS	1.5	196	191	68	IV	63	0.5	NA	0.002 @ 60 min (Q_B= 200, Q_F= 15 ml/min)
5		APS-15DSplus			197	193	66	IV	51	0.5		
6		VPS-15HA			196	190	62	IV	63	0.5		
7		APS-15E			190	183	74	V	66	3.0		0.008 @ 60 min (Q_B= 200, Q_F= 15 ml/min)
8		APS-15EX			194	191	74	V	66	4.0		
9		APS-15EL			190	181	72	V	64	1.0		0.004 @ 60 min (Q_B= 200, Q_F= 15 ml/min)
10		APS-15MD			187	175	58	IV	52	0.2		0.002 @ 60 min (Q_B= 200, Q_F= 15 ml/min)

11	Kawasumi Laboratories, Inc.	KF-15C	EVAL	1.5	181	165	18	II	11.1	3.0	NA	0.04 @ 60 min (Q_B = 200, Q_F = 15 ml/min)
		Notes: Clearance (urea nitrogen, creatinine) in aqueous solution, TMP = 13.3 kPa (100 mm Hg). Ultrafiltration coefficient and s.c. (albumin) with bovine blood										
12		kf-m15		1.5	175	155	17	II	11.5	2.0	NA	0.03 @ 60 min (Q_B = 200, Q_F = 15 ml/min)
		Notes: Clearance (urea nitrogen, creatinine) in aqueous solution, ultrafiltration flow rate per unit surface area Q_F/A_o = 10 ml/min/m^2. Ultrafiltration coefficient and s.c. (albumin) with bovine blood										
13		KF-15		1.5	179	157	NA	II	8.7	1.5	NA	0.02 @ 60 min (Q_B = 200, Q_F = 15 ml/min)
		Notes: Clearance (urea nitrogen, creatinine) in aqueous solution, TMP = 13.3 kPa (100 mm Hg) Ultrafiltration coefficient and s.c. (albumin) with bovine blood										
14		RENAK PS-1.3	PS	1.3	191	183	58	IV	75	NA	NA	<0.01 @ 60 min (Q_B = 200, Q_F = 13 ml/min)
15	Nikkiso Co.	FLX-15GW	PEPA	1.5	190	NA	52	IV	40	1.0	NA	NA
		Notes: k_{UF} bovine blood (not applicable to [b, d])										
16		FDX-150GW		1.5	190	NA	52	IV	50	0.5	NA	NA
17		FDY-150GW					65	IV	52	1.0		
18		FDY-15GW					71	V	51	0.3		
19		FDZ-15					72	V	81	1.5		
20	JMS Co.	BP-N150	PES	1.5	192	183	75	V	109	2.0	1.0 ± 0.3	0.01 @ 60 min (Q_B = 200, Q_F = 15 ml/min)
		Notes: Bovine plasma TP 6.0 ± 0.5 g/dl Bovine blood Ht = 32 ± 2 %, TP = 6.0 ± 0.5 g/dl										

No.	Maker	Japanese brand name	Main material of the membrane	Surface area A_o, m^2	Clearance, ml/min[B,C]			Class according to the Japanese reimburse-ment system	Ultrafiltration coefficient k_{UF}[B,D] ml/h/mm Hg	Albumin loss		
					urea nitro-gen	creati-nine	β_2-MG			targeted value per 4-hour clinical treatment, g	in vitro 4-hour dialysis experiment, g	*s.c.* @ XXX min (Q_B = XXX, Q_F = YY, ml/min) [–]
21	Nipro Co.	FB-150FH eco	PES	1.5	196	NA	65	IV	85.6	6.0	6.0	NA
22		FB-150Uβ eco			195		55	IV	76.9	0.5	0.5	
23		FB-150Pβ eco			195		53	IV	74.8	0.3	0.3	
24		FB-150UHβ eco			196		75	V	74.8	4.0	4.0	
25		PES-15Eα eco			194		65	IV	57.9	0.5	0.5	
26		PES-15Gα eco			194		60	IV	55.2	0.3	0.3	
27		PES-15Sα eco			196		75	V	77.4	1.5	1.5	
28		PES-15SEαeco			196		73	V	77.0	1.0	1.0	
29		PES-15Dα eco			196		77	V	86.9	3.0	3.0	
30	Toray Co.	BK-1.6U	PMMA	1.6	177	NA	51	III	27	NA	NA	0.006 @ over 30 min (Q_B = 200 ml/min)
		Notes: Bovine blood was used in the measure-ment of s.c. albumin										
31		BG-1.6U	PMMA	1.6	189		55	IV	43	NA	NA	0.003 @ over 30 min (Q_B = 200 ml/min)
32		BG-1.6PQ			187		55	IV	59			0.009 @ over 30 min (Q_B = 200 ml/min)

33	TS-1.6SL	PS	191	59	IV	54	0.003 @ over 30 min (Q_B = 200 ml/min)
34	TS-1.6UL		189	61	IV	77	0.006 @ over 30 min (Q_B = 200 ml/min)
35	TS-1.6PLX		193	76	V	198	0.011 @ over 30 min (Q_B = 200 ml/min)
36	NV-16S		192	60	IV	94	0.003 @ over 30 min (Q_B = 200 ml/min)
37	NV-16U		189	68	IV	116	0.005 @ over 30 min (Q_B = 200 ml/min)
38	NV-16X		193	76	V	122	0.008 @ over 30 min (Q_B = 200 ml/min)

[A] All data were taken by the producing company.
[B] Plasma was used as a pseudo blood in the experiment.
[C] Measurement of clearances was performed under the following flow conditions, i.e., blood flow rate Q_B = 200 ml/min, dialysis fluid flow rate Q_D = 500 ml/min, and ultrafiltration flow rate per unit surface area Q_F/A_o = 10 ml/min/m^2, unless otherwise specified.
[D] Ultrafiltration coefficient was calculated considering the effect of oncotic pressure.
[E] Values, especially k_{UF} and *s.c.* for albumin, vary drastically in view of the reproducibility from laboratory to laboratory.
[F] Listed models are the ones, the surface area of which is the closest to 1.5 m^2.
[G] Classifications of dialyzers (class I to class V) are based on the clearances for β_2- that are normalized to 1.5 m^2 by using the classic performance evaluation equation if necessary.

Classes	Clearances for β_2-MG ml/min
Class I	<10
Class II	≤10 <30
Class III	≤30 <50
Class IV	≤50 <70
Class V	≤70

Author Index

Subject Index